Psychological Interventions in Mental Health Nursing

Psychological Interventions in Mental Health Nursing

Grahame Smith

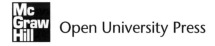 Open University Press

Open University Press
McGraw-Hill Education
McGraw-Hill House
Shoppenhangers Road
Maidenhead
Berkshire
England
SL6 2QL

email: enquiries@openup.co.uk
world wide web: www.openup.co.uk

and Two Penn Plaza, New York, NY 10121-2289, USA

First published 2012

A catalogue record of this book is available from the British Library

ISBN-13: 9780335244164 (pb)
ISBN-10: 0335244165 (pb)
e-ISBN: 9780335244171

Library of Congress Cataloging-in-Publication Data
CIP data has been applied for

Typeset by Aptara Inc., India
Printed in the UK by Bell and Bain Ltd, Glasgow

The **McGraw-Hill** Companies

Contents

Contributors

Denise Aspinall is a senior lecturer in mental health nursing at the Faculty of Health and Applied Social Sciences at Liverpool John Moores University. She is also programme lead for the Personality Disorders programme and the BSc Pre-registration Mental Health Nursing programme.

May Baker is a senior lecturer in mental health nursing at the Faculty of Health and Applied Social Sciences at Liverpool John Moores University. Her interests are dual diagnosis, alcohol use and motivational interviewing.

Ged Carney is a learning disability nurse at Merseycare NHS Trust, who has experience of working with people who have complex needs. He has previously worked in a senior clinical position providing services for people with mental health problems.

John Harrison is a senior lecturer in mental health nursing at Liverpool John Moores University, who has worked with children with mental health problems and as a community nurse with the British Army. His interests include attitudes towards eating disorders in the young and the use of light therapy in agitation.

Paula Kennedy is a senior lecturer in mental health nursing in the Faculty of Health and Applied Social Sciences at Liverpool John Moores University, with interests in systemic family therapy, and leadership and management.

Deborah Knott is a senior lecturer in mental health nursing, and admissions tutor in the Faculty of Health and Applied Social Sciences at Liverpool John Moores University. Her interests include communication skills, working with long-term conditions and solution-focused approaches.

Denise Parker is a senior lecturer in mental health nursing, and programme leader for the Dementia Care programme in the Faculty of Health and Applied Social Sciences at Liverpool John Moores University. Her interests include dementia care, the context of mental health care, and research methods.

Karen Rea is a senior lecturer in mental health nursing and programme lead for the IAPT programme at Liverpool John Moores University. She is a registered cognitive behavioural therapy practitioner who has extensive clinical experience in the areas of community learning disability services and community and in-patient mental health.

James Ridley is a learning disability nurse at Merseycare NHS Trust; he is a member of the Liverpool community learning disability team. He is interested in the analysis of complex behaviours and how this impacts on individuals throughout their life and how services respond.

Rebecca Rylance is a mental health nurse practitioner at 5 Boroughs Partnership NHS Foundation Trust. She has an academic and research interest in physical health and well-being among people with mental health issues, and a clinical interest in suicide prevention and self-harm reduction.

Peter Simpson is a mental health lecturer/practitioner at 5 Boroughs Partnership NHS Foundation Trust. He works in the learning and development team with interests in risk assessment and risk management, suicide prevention and the management of self-injury.

Grahame Smith is a mental health nurse with extensive experience within acute mental health in-patient settings, who has interests in descriptive psychopathology, history of mental health care, and mental health ethics. He is a principal lecturer in the Faculty of Health and Applied Social Sciences at Liverpool John Moores University.

Lisa Woods is a senior lecturer and the professional lead for mental health nursing at Liverpool John Moores University. She has a range of clinical experiences across community mental health and day service settings; her areas of interest include child and adolescent mental health, psychological therapies and public mental health.

An introduction to psychological interventions

Grahame Smith

Chapter aim and objectives

Aim

- To provide a contextualized overview of the book.

Objectives

- To define the term psychological interventions and its relationship to collaboration, risk and making sense of the evidence.
- To provide a chapter-by-chapter overview.

Psychological interventions in context

This book is primarily aimed at pre-registration mental health nursing students, though aspects of the book will be just as useful to other health-care students or professionals who are looking for specific information about how to care for individuals with mental health needs. Qualified mental health nurses as well as other mental health professionals who want to want to refresh their knowledge-base may also find this book useful.

The core idea for this book stems from recognizing mental health nurses' increasing use of psychological therapies within their practice (Department of Health, 2006a; 2006b; Callaghan, 2009; Norman and Ryrie, 2009). So why not write a book about a psychological therapy or about a number of psychological therapies rather than focusing on a more nebulous topic such as psychological interventions? Well this book is based on the premise that the core work of the mental health nurse is to deliver a variety of psychological interventions, some of which are framed by a specific therapeutic approach but most are eclectically taken from a number of therapeutic approaches (Paley and Shapiro, 2001; Department of Health, 2006a; 2006b; Callaghan, 2009). This eclectic approach to the use of psychological interventions starts during the mental health nurse's pre-qualifying journey and usually continues throughout a mental health nurse's career, though of course some mental health nurses may go on to specialize in the use of a specific psychological therapy (Paley and Shapiro, 2001; Department of Health, 2006b). This book is, therefore, intended to assist the pre-registration mental health nurse in this developmental journey by providing a good grounding in the use of psychological interventions (Department of Health, 2006b; Callaghan, 2009; Nursing and Midwifery Council, 2010). It will signpost to a specific psychological therapy where appropriate, but it is not a replacement for the number of excellent texts available for mental health nurses that deal with the delivery of a specific psychological therapy.

What is a psychological intervention? For the purposes of this book a psychological intervention is broadly understood as a mental health nursing intervention which is underpinned by psychological methods and theory. It also has the intention of improving biopsychosocial functioning and it is usually delivered via a therapeutically structured relationship (Paley and Shapiro, 2001; Hurley and Rankin, 2008; Thompson et al., 2008; Department of Health, 2006a; Callaghan, 2009; Gournay, 2009).

It is important to note that these interventions should be clinically effective, where possible evidenced based, and they should also consider the values and meanings that are inherent within the therapeutic relationship (Bracken and Thomas, 2005; Callaghan and Crawford, 2009; Cooper, 2009; Playle and Bee, 2009). To take this considered approach the mental health nurse must acknowledge that their professional understanding of a service user's experience is not necessarily the same as the service user's understanding of their experience, and that by doing this the nurse creates an opportunity to preserve rather than potentially lose the true meaning of the service user's experience (Merleau-Ponty, [1945]1962; Austin, 1968; Brimblecombe et al., 2007; Simpson, 2009).

The following two extracts from a journal by Mary O'Hagan (1996) kept during her time on an in-patient mental health unit illustrates this point. The first extract describes a specific experience that Mary had at the start of her stay on the unit, and the second extract is a mental health professional's interpretation of that experience, which was accrued by Mary from both the medical and nursing notes.

Mary's experience: 'I stand alone, unable to move inside a dark bubble. I have no face or hands or feet. My veins are broken and my blood has nowhere to travel. Outside the bubble it is day. A rainbow appears but I cannot see it. I remain in the bubble, broken and hidden from life around me' (O'Hagan, 1996: 199). The mental health professional's interpretation: 'Mary has an inadequate and confused sense of identity. She also has a long-standing picture of being an isolate; tending to live in her own world and always finding it difficult to fit in. In this way she presents a schizoid personality picture' (O'Hagan, 1996: 199).

The differences can clearly be seen to have arisen from the mental health professional's need to find a 'professional meaning' and in doing so they have 'over-analysed' and moved substantially away from 'Mary's' meaning (Merleau-Ponty, [1945]1962; O'Hagan, 1996; Bracken and Thomas, 2005; Hamilton and Roper, 2006). Once Mary had identified the differences she made this point: 'Several years later I read what they had written about me and I couldn't believe that my journal and their notes referred to the same person and events. The incongruity between these two accounts of my mental distress is disturbing and I believe exposes the fundamental reason why mental health services so often fail to help people' (O'Hagan, 1996: 199).

To avoid falling into this trap, the mental health nurse needs to be 'aware of their underlying assumptions' about the service user's story, which is why being collaborative and person-centred is such an important part of the therapeutic relationship (Bracken and Thomas, 2005; Hamilton and Roper, 2006; Department of Health, 2006a; Simpson, 2009).

The importance of collaboration

As previously highlighted, one of the difficulties inherent within the therapeutic relationship is that the mental health nurse, in their search for professional understanding, can fall into the trap of reconstructing meanings to the point where an agréed true meaning is lost (Merleau-Ponty, [1945]1962). As a further example the experience of hearing voices may have the meaning for an individual that 'God is communicating with them', but for the mental health nurse the meaning of these 'voices' is at first shaped by professional understanding such as a medical diagnosis and second by the professional 'helper's' need to find a remedy (Watkins, 1998; Simpson, 2009). In essence the individual's experience is being 'reconstructed' to fit the mental health nurse's professional understanding, motivations and values (Bertram and Stickley, 2005). This can in turn create a potential divide between the individual's meaning of their experiences of mental distress and the mental health nurse's 'reconstructed' understanding. However, for the relationship to be fruitful this divide will need to be managed (Hamilton and Roper, 2006; Wilkin, 2006; Simpson, 2009).

Understanding different values is part and parcel of the mental health nurse's role, although sometimes this can be clouded by the belief in a single objective truth, a belief that emanates from an evidence-based practice approach (Bracken and Thomas, 2005; Simpson, 2009). Key to exploring other truths is for the mental health nurse to work collaboratively within the therapeutic relationship (Bracken and Thomas, 2005; Simpson, 2009). A starting place for collaborative working is to encourage the exploration of multiple or plural truths by empowering the mental health service user to 'become the authors of their own stories' and at the same time the mental health nurse should take the position of being interested in a way that is similar to 'reading a novel for the first time' (Bracken and Thomas, 2005; Simpson, 2009). By taking this viewpoint the mental health service user's narrative becomes real and the mental health service user's experience is understood as something unique rather than a written and static case history based on objectifying nursing problems (Bracken and Thomas, 2005; Martinez, 2009).

This narrative approach gives the mental health nurse the opportunity to open themselves up to being more thoughtful about the interventions they deliver within the therapeutic relationship; interventions can then be formulated through a collaborative understanding rather than being based on an 'illusion of understanding' (Bracken and Thomas, 2005; Simpson, 2009). This illusion of understanding can be seen in the case where a mental health service user views their 'voice-hearing' as part of their spiritual development and, as such, a positive experience, despite taking time adapting to this change in their life, but this experience could be potentially reconstructed by the mental health nurse as appearing negative (Watkins, 1998). Negativity may be transmitted through the use of common psychological terms such as not coping (negative) rather than focusing on the positive element of the mental health service user's story (Romme, 1993; Bracken and Thomas, 2005).

Using a narrative approach also gives the mental health nurse the scope to understand the complex ethical nature of delivering psychological interventions within the mental health field (Martinez, 2009). Mental health nurses have the sanctioned power, where risk indicates to use coercion, to restrict the freedoms of a mental health service user, which can impact upon the therapeutic relationship and any subsequent psychological interventions that are delivered (Bracken and Thomas, 2005; Roberts, 2005).

The risk dimension

The therapeutic relationship within the mental health field, unlike most health-care relationships, tends to be both the medium for treatment as well as, in most cases, the main treatment itself (Radden, 2002; Department of Health, 2006a; O'Carroll and Park, 2007; Hurley, 2009). For the therapeutic relationship to be effective it has to follow a process which is built upon the mental health nurse using both reason and emotion not as separate entities, but as entities working in unison (Department of Health, 2006a; 2006b; Simpson, 2009). On this basis the mental health nurse might reason that a core statutory component of the therapeutic relationship is to manage risk. However, there may also be an emotional context that needs to be taken into account, such as making difficult emotional decisions around managing risk through temporarily restricting liberty (Roberts, 2005; Eales, 2009). In this type of situation the effective mental health nurse needs to be 'emotionally responsive' both to how the mental health service user is experiencing their mental distress and also to how the mental health service user feels about the restriction of their liberty (Roberts, 2004).

Being able to restrict a person's liberty means that the mental health nurse has society-sanctioned power, which will impact upon the collaborative element of the therapeutic relationship and, in turn, needs to be recognized and understood by the mental health nurse (Roberts, 2004; 2005). A starting place to understand the impact of power is to look at the role of the mental illness label. The concept of mental illness is conceptually controversial but, even so, once an individual is labelled mentally ill then, if required, the mental health nurse has the power given by society to control that individual (Radden, 2002; Roberts, 2004; 2005). This approach emanates from the view that an individual who is labelled mentally ill has an increased potential to exhibit diminished judgement and because of this they are then perceived as being more risky or dangerous than the 'average person' in society (Radden, 2002; Eales, 2009).

The effect of this view upon mental health nursing practice is that mental health nurses, when working with individuals who are labelled as mentally ill, have to then consider risk containment and risk minimization as a central approach (Duffy et al., 2004; Roberts, 2005; Eales, 2009). In terms of the therapeutic relationship this means that even though it is intended to be collaborative and person-centred this intention is dependent on risk. So where a mental health service user's behaviour is deemed to be 'low risk' the approach can be more collaborative. It becomes more difficult however in the case of working with high-risk behaviours such as self-harm and harm to others

(Roberts, 2005; Perraud et al., 2006; Wilkin, 2006). At the higher level of risk the mental health nurse would still be empathetic and collaborative but they would also be looking to control any perceived risk and, if required, the mental health practitioner would have the power to fully control the situation, which could mean taking a mental health service user's freedoms away (Duffy et al., 2004; Roberts, 2005; O'Carroll and Park, 2007; Eales, 2009).

Identifying, predicting and managing risk is an important part of the mental health nurse's role. The nurse needs to use both reasoning and person-centred skills to collaboratively formulate the best way to mange the presenting risk (Duffy et al., 2004; Eales, 2009). During this process the nurse will be required to use different forms of knowledge to make sense of the evidence, such as scientific knowledge, and also personal or tacit knowledge (Welsh and Lyons, 2001).

Making sense of the evidence

A mental health nurse's knowledge is developed in a number of ways. The basic foundation of their knowledge is based on their professional training where different forms of knowledge are introduced. In the main this emanates from the human and physical sciences (Welsh and Lyons, 2001; Department of Health, 2006a; 2006b). This knowledge is further developed into 'ways of knowing', such as scientific, naturalistic, personal and ethical (Carper, 1978). Added to these layers of knowledge is the nurse's own experiences of being a practitioner which, in turn, subsequently shapes their practice and their understanding of their practice (Welsh and Lyons, 2001; Hardy et al., 2002).

Scientific evidence is a key form of knowledge used in mental health nursing practice, which is referred to as evidence-based practice (Callaghan and Crawford, 2009). It is recognized that the best evidence is that which is based on the 'systematic review of randomized controlled trials', but for this evidence to be effective it has to also be situated within the mental health nurse–service user relationship, reflecting the specific needs of the mental health service user (Welsh and Lyons, 2001; Callaghan and Crawford, 2009). On this basis, the implication is that scientific knowledge may struggle to provide an 'established truth', therefore there is a need to complement scientific evidence with situational-type evidence (Benner and Tanner, 1987; Welsh and Lyons, 2001; Franks, 2004). Certainly having a 'one fits all' approach can be seen as a limited way of understanding mental distress; a better understanding can be generated through integrating understandings, especially as a service user's experience can have multiple meanings (Carper, 1978; Lakeman, 2006).

One way in which mental health nurses complement scientific knowledge is through using naturalistic knowledge or tacit knowledge (Benner and Tanner, 1987; Welsh and Lyons, 2001; Department of Health, 2006a). This tacit realm of knowledge, or what has become called 'tacit knowledge', is also known originally via the work of Polanyi (1958) as the 'tacit component of knowledge'. Tacit knowledge can be seen as implicit knowledge which is based on personal experience. It has an automatic feel to it, in that a person may act effectively but they may not be aware of acting – for example, driving your car home safely but not being able to recall the journey

(Carlsson, et al., 2000). Welsh and Lyons (2001: 301) further describe tacit knowledge as 'a synthesis of the formal knowledge and clinical expertise which nurses have accumulated over the years'. One of the difficulties of using tacit knowledge on its own is that it often is seen as not being scientific and therefore must be based on guesswork (Benner and Tanner, 1987; Welsh and Lyons, 2001). Some of these negative views arise from the stance that the best professional knowledge can only be scientific; one of the weaknesses of this absolute view is that it does not account for knowledge that is based on experience and expert understanding, which is the realm of the expert mental health nurse (Schon, 1983; Benner and Tanner, 1987; Welsh and Lyons, 2001).

Closs (1994) makes the point that although science is about 'understanding the world' it will 'not produce absolute truths' especially in relation to 'human behaviours and emotions'. Closs goes on to say that science is not the only 'useful knowledge' which can be used by nurses; more subjective ways of knowing, such as intuition, can be just as useful. On this basis it is important to recognize that the use of tacit knowledge in mental health nursing is not seen as a replacement for scientific knowledge; it is also seen as a way to complement and enhance the use of scientific knowledge (Welsh and Lyons, 2001; Callaghan and Crawford, 2009).

An overview of the book

As previously mentioned, this book has been written primarily for pre-registration mental health nursing students, so the chapters of this book are organized in a way that is intended to support the student's learning journey. This book is not a substitute for learning by fully engaging with the theory and practice elements of your programme; instead it focuses on helping you to make sense of those learning experiences that relate to the use of psychological interventions (Arnold and Thompson, 2009).

Generally each chapter in the book will build on the points made in this introductory chapter, paying careful attention to the importance of collaboration, the risk dimension and making sense of the evidence. There is an emphasis on capturing the service user's narrative by taking a scenario-based approach. Also the chapters have been organized in such a way that there is a sense of consistency if you want to read the text from cover to cover and a sense of individuality if you just want to dip in to the chapters on a stand-alone basis. It is important to re-state that although this book provides a good grounding in the use of psychological interventions, it is not a psychological therapies text. It will, where required, signpost to a specific psychological therapy and any relevant clinical guidelines or any planned changes to those guidelines (see the review process for DSM V via the American Psychiatric Association website) (Department of Health, 2006a; 2006b; Callaghan, 2009; Callaghan and Crawford, 2009).

You will find that every chapter will state its aim(s) and objectives, giving a sense of what it is about. A scenario approach will be used in each chapter to demonstrate how this knowledge can be applied to practice. This approach does not stop you from applying your own experiences to test this knowledge; indeed this is encouraged as part of the supervised process of you critically thinking and reflecting about your practice experiences (Department of Health, 2006b; Nursing and Midwifery Council, 2010). You may find that you do not agree with a given approach and on this basis you are further encouraged to undertake supervised research to support your views (Arnold and Thompson, 2009). Each chapter will then provide a summary of the key points and a quick quiz which will give you the opportunity to interact further with both the chapter and with your learning (Arnold and Thompson, 2009).

In summary, the first two chapters will provide you with a working definition of psychological interventions that is utilized throughout the text; a good grounding in how risk is managed within the mental health field, paying particular attention to psychological interventions; and how the use of communication skills provides a fundamental basis for the delivery of these interventions. The next eight chapters are the core of the text, both describing and analysing how psychological interventions, within the field of mental health are used in a variety of conditions and contexts. Chapter 11 pays particular attention to the ethical context of psychological interventions. It does not specifically explore the use of legal frameworks but its approach to a moral reasoning process ensures that it is compatible with the use of these frameworks. The concluding chapter focuses on tying the book's themes together; it also provides some insights into the newly qualified mental health nurse's future use of psychological intervention, especially in relation to the journey towards expert practice.

Summary of the key points

Mental health nurses commonly use psychological interventions which may or may not be formally framed by a specific psychological therapy.

To be clinically effective psychological interventions need to be framed by the respective service user's narrative.

Mental health nurses need to recognize the coercive element present within their practice.

It is important for mental health nurses when making decisions to consider all forms of knowledge and not to rely on one form alone.

This book is primarily intended to assist the student's learning journey.

Quick quiz

1   Define psychological interventions.
2   Why is collaboration important?
3   How do you pay attention to the service user's narrative?
4   Why is the therapeutic relationship between the mental health nurse and the mental health service user potentially different than other health-care relationships?
5   What impact does the issue of risk have on the therapeutic relationship?
6   Describe two forms of knowledge that mental health nurses use.
7   What is tacit knowledge?

References

Arnold, L. and Thompson, K. (2009) Learning to learn through real world inquiry in the virtual paradigm, *Journal of Learning & Teaching Research*, 1: 6–33.

Austin, J.L. (1968) A plea for excuses, in A.R. White (ed.) *The Philosophy of Action*. Oxford: Oxford University Press.

Benner, P. and Tanner, C. (1987) Clinical judgment: how expert nurses use intuition, *American Journal of Nursing*, 87(1): 23–31.

Bertram, G. and Stickley, T. (2005) Mental health nurses, promoters of inclusion or perpetuators of exclusion, *Journal of Psychiatric and Mental Health Nursing*, 12: 387–95.

Bracken, P. and Thomas, P. (2005) *Postpsychiatry: Mental Health in a Postmodern World*. Oxford: Oxford University Press.

Brimblecombe, N., Tingle, A., Tunmore, R. and Murrell, T. (2007) Implementing holistic practices in mental health nursing: a national consultation, *International Journal of Nursing Studies*, 44: 339–48.

Callaghan, P. (2009) Introduction: mental nursing past, present, and future, in P. Callaghan, J. Playle and L. Cooper (eds) *Mental Health Nursing Skills*. Oxford: Oxford University Press.

Callaghan, P. and Crawford, P. (2009) Evidence-based mental health nursing practice, in P. Callaghan, J. Playle and L. Cooper (eds) *Mental Health Nursing Skills*. Oxford: Oxford University Press.

Carlsson, G., Dahlberg, K. and Drew, N. (2000) Encountering violence and aggression in mental health nursing: a phenomenological study of tacit caring knowledge, *Issues in Mental Health Nursing*, 21: 533–45.

Carper, B.A. (1978) Fundamental patterns of knowing in nursing, *Advances in Nursing Science*, 1(1): 13–23.

Closs, S.J. (1994) What's so awful about science? *Nurse Researcher*, 2(2): 69–83.

Cooper, L. (2009) Values-based mental health nursing practice, in P. Callaghan, J. Playle and L. Cooper (eds) *Mental Health Nursing Skills*. Oxford: Oxford University Press.

Department of Health (2006a) *From Values to Action: The Chief Nursing Officer's Review of Mental Health Nursing*. London, Department of Health.

Department of Health (2006b) *Best Practice Competencies and Capabilities for Pre-registration Mental Health Nurses in England: The Chief Nursing Officer's Review of Mental Health Nursing*. London: Department of Health.

Duffy, D., Doyle, M. and Ryan, T. (2004) Risk assessment and management in acute mental health care, in M. Harrison, D. Howard and D. Mitchell (eds) *Acute Mental Health Nursing: From Acute Concerns to the Capable Practitioner*. London: Sage.

Eales, S. (2009) Risk assessment and management, in P. Callaghan, J. Playle and L. Cooper (eds) *Mental Health Nursing Skills*. Oxford: Oxford University Press.

Franks, V. (2004) Evidence-based uncertainty in mental health nursing, *Journal of Psychiatric and Mental Health Nursing*, 11: 99–105.

Gournay, K. (2009) Psychosocial interventions, in R. Newell and K. Gournay (eds) *Mental Health Nursing: An Evidence-based Approach*, 2nd edn. London: Churchill Livingstone.

Hamilton, B. and Roper, C. (2006) Troubling 'insight': power and possibilities in mental health care, *Journal of Psychiatric and Mental Health Nursing*, 13: 416–22.

Hardy, S., Garbett. R., Titchen. A. and Manley. K. (2002) Exploring nursing expertise: nurses talk nursing, *Nursing Inquiry*, 9: 196–202.

Hurley, J. (2009) A qualitative study of mental health nurse identities: many roles, one profession, *International Journal of Mental Health Nursing*, 18: 383–90.

Hurley, J. and Rankin, R. (2008) As mental health nursing roles expand, is education expanding mental health nurses? An emotionally intelligent view towards preparation for psychological therapies and relatedness, *Nursing Inquiry*, 15(3): 199–205.

Lakeman, R. (2006) An anxious profession in an age of fear, *Journal of Psychiatric and Mental Health Nursing*, 13: 395–400.

Martinez, R. (2009) Narrative ethics, in S. Bloch and S.A. Green (eds) *Psychiatric Ethics*, 4th edn. Oxford: Oxford University Press.

Merleau-Ponty, M. ([1945]1962) The body as expression and speech, *The Phenomenology of Perception*. Trans. C. Smith, 1962. London: Routledge.

Norman, I. and Ryrie, I. (2009) Mental health nursing: origins and traditions, in I. Norman and I. Ryrie (eds) *The Art and Science of Mental Health Nursing: A Textbook of Principles and Practice*, 2nd edn. Maidenhead: McGraw-Hill.

Nursing and Midwifery Council (2010) *Standards for Pre-registration Nursing Education*. London: Nursing and Midwifery Council.

O'Carroll, M. and Park, A. (2007) *Essential Mental Health Nursing Skills*. London: Mosby.

O'Hagan, M. (1996) Two accounts of mental distress, in J. Reynolds, R. Muston, T. Heller, J. Leach, M. McCormick, J. Wallcraft and M. Walsh (eds) *Mental Health Still Matters*. Basingstoke: Palgrave Macmillan.

Paley, G. and Shapiro, D. (2001) Evidence-based psychological interventions in mental health nursing, *Nursing Times*, 97(3): 34.

Perraud, S., Delaney, K.R., Carlson-Sabelli, L., Johnson, M.E., Shephard, R. and Paun, O. (2006) Advanced practice psychiatric mental health nursing, finding our core: the therapeutic relationship in 21st century, *Perspectives in Psychiatric Care*, 42(4): 215–26.

Playle, J. and Bee, P. (2009) Service user's expectations and views of mental health nurses, in P. Callaghan, J. Playle and L. Cooper (eds) *Mental Health Nursing Skills*. Oxford: Oxford University Press.

Polanyi, M. (1958) *Personal Knowledge: Towards a Post-Critical Philosophy*. Chicago, IL: University of Chicago Press.

Radden, J. (2002) Notes towards a professional ethics for psychiatry, *Australian and New Zealand Journal of Psychiatry*, 36: 52–9.

Roberts, M. (2004) Psychiatric ethics: a critical introduction for mental health nurses, *Journal of Psychiatric and Mental Health Nursing*, 11: 583–88.

Roberts, M. (2005) The production of the psychiatric subject: power, knowledge and Michel Foucault, *Nursing Philosophy*, 6: 33–42.

Romme, M. (1993) Rehabilitating voice-hearers, in T. Heller, J. Reynolds, R. Gomm, R. Muston and S. Pattison (eds) *Mental Health Matters*. London: Macmillan.

Schon, D. (1983) From technical rationality to reflection-in-action, in R. Harrison, F. Reeve, A. Hanson and J. Clarke (eds) *Supporting Lifelong Learning: Perspectives on Learning*. London: RoutledgeFalmer.

Simpson, A. (2009) Working in partnership, in P. Callaghan, J. Playle and L. Cooper (eds) *Mental Health Nursing Skills*. Oxford: Oxford University Press.

Thompson, P., Lang, L. and Annells, M. (2008) A systematic review of the effectiveness of in-home community nurse led interventions for the mental health of older persons, *Journal of Clinical Nursing*, 17: 1419–27.

Watkins, J. (1998) *Hearing Voices: A Common Human Experience*. Melbourne: Hill of Content.

Welsh, I. and Lyons, C.M. (2001) Evidence-based care and the case for intuition and tacit knowledge in clinical assessment and decision making in mental health nursing practice: an empirical contribution to the debate, *Journal of Psychiatric and Mental Health Nursing*, 8: 299–305.

Wilkin, P. (2006) In search of the true self: a clinical journey through the vale of soul-searching, *Journal of Psychiatric and Mental Health Nursing*, 13: 12–18.

1   Psychological interventions and managing risk

Rebecca Rylance and Peter Simpson

Chapter aim and objectives

Aim

*   To provide an overview of the risk assessment process and to explore the psychological interventions that can be utilized when enabling service users to manage risk.

Objectives

*   To identify the components of a typical mental health clinical risk assessment and recognize the different approaches to the assessment of risk.
*   To identify protective factors.
*   To analyse how the therapeutic use of self relates to the risk assessment process.
*   To recognize the tensions that exist between duties concerning safeguarding and the therapeutic nurse–patient relationship.

Introduction

Clinical risk assessment and its subsequent management is a necessary and requisite skill for all mental health nurses (Pratt, 2001) and is a field-specific competency identified by the Nursing and Midwifery Council (NMC) standards for pre-registration nursing education (NMC, 2010). Furthermore, clinical risk assessment is a key feature of clinical governance (DH, 2006; NHS Quality Improvement Scotland, 2010). Broadly speaking, risk in mental health is defined as the likelihood of an event happening with potentially harmful consequences for self and/or others (Morgan, 2000). Risk assessment is the gathering of specific information about an individual, which, when subsequently analysed, enables practitioners to anticipate possible future change. Thus risk management facilitates the opportunity for practitioners to intervene in a positive way that empowers service users and manages risks (DH, 2007). This chapter will explore the common risks that exist among people with mental illness, and will examine the therapeutic strategies that may be utilized to assess, manage and minimize risk in a meaningful way.

To ensure that the ideas, notions and concepts considered in this chapter have a practical value the following scenario will be used and developed throughout the chapter.

SCENARIO

The Primary Care Team have asked you to assess a 51-year-old male, Mike. Mike got made redundant from his executive position in a large pharmaceutical company several months ago. His wife is worried about him as he is spending his time sitting at home, shouting at the children and making no effort to search for a new job. He has withdrawn from his social circle and social activity, which consisted of weekly golf with his work colleagues, preferring instead to stay at home and drink whisky. He doesn't regard his alcohol consumption as significant, claiming to consume three bottles a week, which helps him to sleep. You have been made aware that he has been banned from driving for 12 months for driving under the influence. Before his redundancy, Mike was confident and self-assured and 'took charge' when necessary. On assessment he is extremely irritable and tearful when asked about his redundancy. He claims to have occasional ideas about suicide, claiming that his family would be 'better off without him'.

Over the past decade mental health services have been the subject of a number of notable public inquiries, exposing significant service failures and highlighting the need for mental health nurses to be able to assess and manage clinical risk more effectively. The Christopher Clunis Inquiry (Ritchie et al., 1994) revealed a tendency by health-care professionals to minimize Christopher Clunis's past violent episodes and a failure to assess his propensity for violence (Coid, 1994; Cooling, 2002). As a result of such inquiries and a shift in government mental health policy (Petch, 2001; Kaliniecka and Shawe-Taylor, 2008), risk assessment and the management of risk behaviour has become a familiar concept in western health care (Crowe and Carlyle, 2003; Webster and Hucker, 2007). Indeed, never before has clinical risk occupied such a critical space in contemporary mental health services. However, the reality of assessing risk in clinical practice is never easy, nor is it an exact science (Green, 2009).

Negative media reporting and the belief held by the general public that psychiatrists and mental health professionals can predict when service users pose a risk to themselves or others (Green, 2009) has served only to perpetuate unrealistic and misinformed expectations about risk (Morgan, 2000). That withstanding, it must be acknowledged that successful clinical risk management protects the public, the professionals and the service user (Green, 2009). However, the literature indicates that there is a general lack of guidance around what to do when risks have been identified (Morgan, 2000). Nevertheless, before we examine the more salient aspects of risk management it is prudent to provide an overview of the risk assessment process.

Risk assessment

Clinical risk assessment is a fundamental part of the Care Programme Approach (CPA) (CPAA, 2008) and should reflect a broad holistic appraisal of a person, taking into account the physical, psychological, sociological and spiritual dimensions (Harrison, 2003). A typical risk assessment should include consideration of the following domains:

- risk to self (suicide, self-harm, neglect)
- risk of harm to others (dangerousness, forensic history)
- risk from others to service user (abuse, harassment, exploitation)
- risk of absconsion
- risk of non-compliance with treatment
- risk of substance misuse.

There is no consensus as to which risk domains should be the priority for mental health workers to address, but there seems to be some agreement that risk behaviours *should* be assessed and, if at all possible, *managed* (Coffey, 2009). Thus, risk assessment involves working with service users and their carers where possible, to weigh up both the potential and the beneficial outcomes by establishing the following:

- How likely is it that the event will happen?
- How soon is it expected to happen?
- How severe is the outcome should it happen?

When considering clinical risks it is useful to acknowledge that there are two essential components, namely static and dynamic factors (DH, 2007; Green, 2009). Static factors are based on facts that generally cannot be changed – for example, social demographics and service-user history. Dynamic factors refer to aspects that can potentially be altered or influenced, such as clinical condition, treatment options and environment of care. The dynamic factors are thought to be more amenable to management and, if they are stable, are often referred to as chronic or stable risk factors (DH, 2007). Risk factors that have the potential to change rapidly are called acute risk factors (DH, 2007). Traditionally risk assessment approaches have been spilt into two broad approaches: actuarial and clinical (Scottish Executive, 2000). However, *The Best Practice in Managing Risk: Principles and Evidence for Best Practice in the Assessment and Management of Risk to Self and Others in Mental Health Services* (DH, 2007) suggests that there are three main approaches to risk assessment: (1) the unstructured clinical approach, (2) the actuarial approach and (3) structured professional judgement (SPJ).

The unstructured clinical approach is generally carried out by a single clinician and is thought to be a somewhat subjective and unsystematic approach to gathering information about risk (DH, 2007). The actuarial approach tends to be more reliable, focusing on a series of set questions often based on statistical data that make risks more or less likely (Scottish Executive, 2000). However, SPJ has gained popularity in recent years and instead of the traditional arbitrary approach of clinicians predicting risk, SPJ is informed by the evidence base. Furthermore, SPJ is not only useful in supporting evidence-based practice, it also facilitates transparency in the decision-making process (Bouch and Marshall, 2005) which is a vital part of clinical audit and governance. SPJ has propelled the development of a number of risk assessment tools such as the Historical Clinical Risk Management-20 (HCR-20) violence risk assessment scheme

(Webster et al., 1997), the Spouse Abuse Risk Assessment (SARA) (Kropp et al., 1995), the Risk of Sexual Violence Protocol (RSVP) (Hart et al., 2003) and the Short-Term Assessment of Risk and Treatability (START) (Webster et al., 2006).

In clinical practice there are a number of risk assessment tools which invariably provide practitioners with prompts to ensure that all aspects of the risk assessment are considered. However, practitioners must not rely solely on such tools (NICE, 2004; Martin, 2006) but instead consider them to complement the risk assessment interview. Indeed, central to the risk assessment process is the clinical interview, where the practitioner can evaluate the service user's current situation and examine how it relates to previous events. This process requires linking the service user's historical information with their presenting circumstances (DH, 2007), taking into consideration the characteristics of their illness and exploring the effective and ineffective interventions from previous episodes of care.

This may require one or a number of practitioners to access the service user's records and to consult with other professionals and agencies. In practice it is also likely that the service user's presentation, coupled with practitioner 'intuition' will contribute significantly to the risk assessment process (Morgan, 2000). That said there is an increasing and opposing body of knowledge that challenges so-called 'professional intuition', and argues that careful and deliberate analysis should be the focus of decisions concerning risk (Lamond and Thompson, 2000). However, Hamm (1988) succinctly proposes that clinical judgement should lie somewhere between intuition and risk analysis.

SCENARIO

In order to assess the risks presented by Mike, it is essential that the mental health nurse systematically considers and explores each of the risk domains. For example, Mike has had a significant change in his circumstances in terms of his redundancy. It would appear that this has affected his mood and behaviour (he is shouting at the children). However, don't assume that his irritability is something new: he may have shouted at the children before he was made redundant. To establish whether this is a new behaviour or increased behaviour you will need to ask him, and possibly involve his wife in your discussions if Mike is agreeable. Your interpersonal skills will assist the establishment of a therapeutic alliance with Mike and will augment your assessment.

Mike may or may not be feeling suicidal despite expressing some suicidal ideas. The only way you can find out how Mike is feeling is to ask him how often he thinks about suicide. If you believe that he is intent on acting on his suicidal thinking, ask him how he intends to do it. Does he have a plan? Does he have the means? Mike held a senior position in a pharmaceutical company; does he have extensive knowledge of drugs? Remember, talking about suicide does not increase the risk, it actually reduces it (NHS Scotland, 2008).

During your assessment, it may become apparent that there are more immediate concerns, for example Mike's alcohol consumption. Could he be withdrawing from alcohol? Is this why he is tearful and irritable? Mike has been charged with a 'driving under the influence' offence, what were the circumstances around this? Was Mike behaving impulsively or recklessly?

The more detailed your risk assessment is, the more informed your prediction of risk will be. In terms of the likelihood of any event happening, it is likely in practice that you will calculate such risks by utilizing a predictive risk assessment tool and possibly your 'gut feeling' to assist with the 'weighing up' of your findings.

In order to address such a delicate balance, it is vital that practitioners also consider the protective factors when assessing risk. There is a considerable amount of evidence that suggests that there are certain ascertainable factors that make risks more or less likely, and have the potential to protect mental health and well-being. Protective factors can be summarized as:

- psychosocial life and coping skills (sense of self-esteem and autonomy, resilience and problem-solving skills)
- meaningful occupation
- family connectedness and or social support; having someone to talk to
- physical activity and health
- hopefulness
- access to resources/services and a mental health professional (McLean et al., 2008).

SCENARIO

In terms of Mike's protective factors, we know that this presenting episode happened recently (he got made redundant several months ago). This may be his first presentation; you need to find out whether there have been other times in his life when he has been in crisis. This will help you to establish previous coping strategies as well as bolstering his confidence that he will get through this. If there have been other episodes, liaise with others – you may be in possession of just one piece of the 'jigsaw'. It is essential that you acquire all the pieces to see the full picture.

Previously Mike held a senior position in a large pharmaceutical company; he used to be 'self-assured' and 'took charge'. Maybe he feels out of control? Explore this with him as this will inform your risk management plan.

Mike has a wife and family, which are generally considered to be protective factors particularly for men (McLean et al., 2008). Up until recently Mike played golf; can you explore if this is an activity that he might wish to pursue again?

Does Mike have anything to look forward to? Family events, weddings, and so on? This will allude to hopefulness, and remember that hopelessness is a critical indicator of suicide (Morgan, 2000).

This is not an exhaustive list but rather a selection of possible protective factors that will require consideration as part of the risk assessment.

In summary, a comprehensive risk assessment will ultimately inform the most ap-propriate level of risk management and the right kind of intervention for a service user (DH, 2007). However, the very dynamic nature of risk demands that mental health practitioners frequently review, evaluate and reassess risks, and duly record amend-ments in the relevant care plans (Harrison, 2003).

Risk management

It follows, then, that risk management is concerned with the development of flexible strategies that prevent an event from occurring; and, where this is not possible, min-imizing the degree of harm (DH, 2007). It must be emphasized that rarely can risk be totally eliminated (NPSA, 2007). Indeed, Harrison (2003) argues that there is no such thing as a risk-free situation and that the risk management plan is more concerned with risk minimization and the prevention of harm or further harm. However, a fun-damental difficulty in managing risk arises as a consequence of balancing the demands placed on mental health services. As Kemshall (2002: 90) has noted, 'Mental health provision is one arena in which needs, rights and risks have long competed.' On the one hand, there is a need to safeguard, to protect and to fulfil a duty of care (Edwards, 1999) while, on the other, there is the general right that people can make their own decisions, act independently and take risks if they so choose.

High-profile public inquiries have concluded that mental health services do need to improve their ability to manage risk in order to protect the public and the vulnerable people in their care (Hally, 1999; Cordall, 2009). Yet these conclusions may also have unintended consequences, with greater and perhaps unrealistic expectations being placed on mental health professionals, who respond by becoming ever more cautious in their assessment of risk (Woods and Kettles, 2009). Ryan (2000) has also argued that these criticisms have led to an increasing emphasis in mental health services on low-frequency/high-impact risks (homicide and suicide) while less attention is paid to the high-frequency/low-impact risks faced by many service users on a daily basis. Aside from the ethical problems that these developments might cause, there are also those who believe that increasingly defensive practice might serve only to increase risks in the longer term (Cordall, 2009) as current thinking on the most effective ways to manage risk is undermined.

It has been suggested that the term 'risk management' should be replaced with alternative phrases such as 'risk enablement', 'risk mitigation' and 'risk benefit assess-ment' (DH, 2010). These alternatives essentially describe the key elements of positive risk management, not the least of which is the recognition that risks cannot always be entirely removed. The Department of Health (2007) has also sought to convey the idea that, to manage risks effectively, practitioners sometimes have to take risks too. In its risk guidance for dementia, for example, the Department of Health (2010) has made explicit the principle that a person should not be prevented from engaging in activities on the basis that they might prove risky, without first considering the benefits of facilitating independent living and decision making. In other words, practitioners are asked to consider the potential risks of independent living but only in light of the costs to the person's quality of life if mental health or other services were to intervene. Furthermore, positive risk management means engaging with the service user and others involved in their care at every stage, as well as recognizing and building on the resources the service user already has available to them, including their own strengths and coping strategies. It also needs to be acknowledged that people have the right to make choices and that sometimes those choices may involve a degree of risk.

The Department of Health (2007) has identified the key principles that should underpin a positive approach to risk management. These principles are:

- Positive risk management as part of a carefully constructed plan is a required competence for all mental health practitioners.
- Risk management should be conducted in a spirit of collaboration and based on a relationship between the service user and their carers that is as trusting as possible.
- Risk management must be built on the recognition of the service user's strengths and should emphasize recovery.

SCENARIO

If you are satisfied that Mike poses no immediate danger to himself or others, you may decide to offer him some 'talking therapies' whether it be counselling or some solution-focused brief therapy to assist with his mood, anxiousness and sleeplessness. You may also decide to make a referral to a primary care 'Lifestyle Team' to offer Mike some help with his alcohol consumption. Furthermore, you may also engage with employment agencies with a view to supporting Mike back to employment. Remember, your risk management plan will be consultative and collaborative, and your role may be primarily supportive. It will specify the actions to take if Mike is unable or unwilling to comply, and all relevant people will be informed.

Of course it is not possible to completely remove risk from people's lives (DH, 2007). Nor is it always possible to reach an agreement on what risks are present, how likely they are to occur and how, if at all, they should be managed. The boundaries between promoting independence and the responsibility to safeguard and protect are often far from clearly defined (Edwards, 1999) and effective risk management often requires a difficult balance to be maintained between safety needs and the needs of the individual service user to make their own choices (see Chapter 11 for further detail) (Cordall, 2009).

At times the need to keep the service user safe or to prevent them from harming others will take priority (Morgan, 2000; DH, 2006), although, even here, the efficacy of the most coercive or intrusive nursing actions, such as physical intervention and close physical observation, remains disputed (Cutcliffe and Barker, 2006; McDonnell and Gallon, 2006). It should also be remembered that the legislative framework within which mental health practitioners operate has an influence. Safeguarding an individual may well be in their best interests, for example, but the least restrictive options available to the practitioner should always be chosen (Mental Capacity Act, 2005). At other times, nursing interventions might focus on 'risk enablement', encouraging the service user to take reasonable risks in order to maintain their independence and quality of life. The decision about where nursing interventions need to be focused is of course determined by the risk assessment.

The way in which risks are managed will be influenced by these and other factors. The nature and severity of the risks present are central to this process, as are the resources available to help maintain safety. Different approaches may well be used depending on whether the individual is residing in an in-patient unit or not. But there is another important factor that will have a significant impact on the decisions made by practitioner, namely the anxiety they might feel about whether they are making the right decision (Morgan, 2000). This anxiety has been acknowledged by the Department of Health (2006), which emphasizes that since risk cannot be eliminated, mental health nurses should consider whether their decisions are defensible. A defensible decision would:

- conform to relevant guidelines
- be based on the best information available
- be documented
- involve informing all relevant people.

Morgan (2000) has also stressed the importance of working collaboratively with other professionals as a means of reducing practitioner anxiety. Sharing information, discussing decisions and offering guidance are all important means of clarifying complex situations, offering support and engendering the confidence required to manage risks positively and effectively.

SCENARIO

The process of risk management is cyclic (Cordall, 2009) with risk assessment being followed by the implementation of appropriate interventions, ongoing monitoring and review, followed by further assessment and changes to the risk management plan if necessary (Doyle, 1999). The cyclical nature of this process underlines the fact that Mike's risks may increase or decrease over time, new risks may emerge, and that the suitability and efficacy of interventions need to be regularly scrutinized and documented.

Minimizing risk

The interventions implemented will vary considerably depending on the individual service user and their environment. A useful way to think about the broad categories of intervention that might be used was suggested by Roberts and Holly (1996). The four levels of intervention they proposed are described as (1) primary, (2) secondary, (3) tertiary and (4) externally imposed. A risk management plan may contain interventions from each of these four levels.

Primary interventions refer to those that are intended to proactively avoid risks occurring. Encouraging and enabling service users to monitor their own symptoms and their relapse or risk indicators would facilitate this process, as would involving other carers in this process. This of course would help to alert service users about when they might need to seek help, rather than waiting until they are in crisis. Positive ways in which the service user manages stress can also be highlighted and incorporated into the overall plan of care. This approach fulfils the requirements of positive risk management, focusing as it does on promoting the ability of the service user to manage their own symptoms. Recovery plans too are a useful way in which these methods can be identified. The Wellness Recovery Action Plan (WRAP) (Copeland, 1997; 2005), for example, contains several useful sections which proactively enable service users to manage risk. Other therapeutic approaches such as problem solving and solution-focused brief therapy (SFBT) also sit well within the contemporary practice of service user empowerment and collaboration (Wiseman, 2003) and can be used to help service users develop new coping strategies or think about new ways of responding to stressful events.

Service-user involvement and the therapeutic relationship are central to the management of risk. Indeed, Ilgen et al. (2009: 249), who explored the therapeutic relationship in relation to the management of suicidal risk, found that a 'collaborative stance in the therapeutic relationship was associated with a significant decrease in suicidal ideation'. A further study (Langan and Lindow, 2004) which examined risk assessment in relation to dangerousness also found that the collaborative relationship between the professional and the service user was highly desirable from the service-user perspective. Thus, it is incumbent upon mental health nurses to initiate and develop therapeutic alliances with service users and their carers.

Of course, not all risks are or can be managed proactively, and secondary-level interventions refer to those that will be implemented should a crisis occur. In essence this is a contingency plan and one that should be prepared in advance, preferably again with service user and carer involvement. If risks occur when a service user's mental health deteriorates, then the plan could be discussed and developed when they are not in crisis. This plan and the service user's wishes, should a crisis occur, can again be documented in their recovery plan. Tertiary-level interventions are those that are necessary to deal with the consequences of a crisis. These may be varied, but the impact of a crisis on the life of the service user and the lives of those around them can be such that they increase the risk of a crisis reoccurring. This needs to be considered and the risks minimized wherever possible. The final level of intervention is those that are externally imposed and are required because of legislation or other guidelines. Those guidelines produced by the Department of Health fall into this category, where there may be a legal requirement to act as a consequence of the 1983 Mental Health Act (amended 2007) or the 2004 Children Act, for example. However, it is always preferable and is considered best practice to utilize primary interventions as far as possible.

Summary of the key points

This chapter has examined the common risks that exist within mental health services, and has discussed the risk assessment and according risk management processes.

Risk management is everyone's business – including the service user (DH, 2007: 25) – however, it is nurses who are often identified as the professional group best placed to ensure the safety of their patients (Currie et al., 2011). It must be accepted that the assessment and management of risk are vital and necessary mental health nursing skills.

It is not always possible to allow service users to take risks when there are perceived harmful or dangerous consequences.

A collaborative therapeutic relationship is imperative throughout the cyclical risk assessment process – that is, risk assessment, risk management, review, risk assessment, and record your findings and amendments.

Quick quiz

1   Risks can be totally eliminated if a comprehensive risk assessment is completed. True/False?
2   Identify the common risks that would be considered as part of a clinical risk assessment.
3   Name three clinical approaches to the assessment of risk.
4   What are protective factors?
5   Which of the following would not be considered a protective factor?
   •   Family support
   •   Meaningful occupation
   •   Poverty
   •   Hopefulness
6   What are the three principles that underpin positive risk management?
7   How do primary, secondary and tertiary interventions differ?

References

Bouch, J. and Marshall, J.J. (2005) Suicide risk: structured professional judgement, *Advances in Psychiatric Treatment*, 11: 84–91.

Care Programme Approach Association (CPAA) (2008) *The CPA and Care Standards Handbook*, 3rd edn. Chesterfield: CPAA.

Coffey, M. (2009) Book reviews, *Journal of Psychiatric and Mental Health Nursing*, 16: 860–4.

Coid, J.W. (1994) The Christopher Clunis Inquiry, *Psychiatric Bulletin*, 18: 449–52.

Cooling, N.J. (2002) Lessons to be learnt from the Christopher Clunis story: a mental health perspective, *Clinical Risk*, 8: 52–5.

Copeland, M.E. (1997) *Wellness Recovery Action Plan*. Dummerston: Peach Press.

Copeland, M.E. (2005) *Wellness Recovery Action Plan: A System for Monitoring, Reducing and Eliminating Uncomfortable or Dangerous Physical Symptoms and Distressing Emotional Feelings or Experiences*. Liverpool: Sefton Recovery Group.

Cordall, J. (2009) Risk assessment and management, in P. Woods and A.M. Kettles (eds) *Risk Assessment and Management in Mental Health Nursing*. Oxford: Blackwell.

Crowe, M. and Carlyle, D. (2003) Deconstructing risk assessment and management in mental health nursing, *Journal of Advanced Nursing*, 43(1): 19–27.

Currie, L., Lecko, C., Gallagher, R. and Sunley, K. (2011) Safety: principle of nursing practice C, *Nursing Standard*, 25(30): 35–7.

Cutcliffe, J.R. and Barker, P. (2006) *Considering the Care of the Suicidal Client and the Case for 'Engagement and Inspiring Hope' or 'Observations'*, in J.R. Cutcliffe and M.F. Ward (eds) *Key Debates in Psychiatric/Mental Health Nursing*. Oxford: Churchill Livingstone.

Department of Health (DH) (2006) *Integrated Governance Handbook: A Handbook for Executives and Non-executives in Healthcare Organisations*. London: Department of Health.

Department of Health (DH) (2007) *Best Practice in Managing Risk: Principles and Evidence for Best Practice in the Assessment and Management of Risk to Self and Others in Mental Health Services*. London: Department of Health.

Department of Health (DH) (2010) *Nothing Ventured, Nothing Gained: Risk Guidance for People with Dementia*. London: Department of Health.

Doyle, M. (1999) Organizational responses to crisis and risk: issues and implications for mental health nurses, in T. Ryan (ed.) *Managing Crisis and Risk in Mental Health Nursing*. Cheltenham: Nelson Thornes.

Edwards, S.D. (1999) Risk assessment in the context of mental health care: some moral considerations, in T. Ryan (ed.) *Managing Crisis and Risk in Mental Health Nursing*. Cheltenham: Nelson Thornes.

Green, B. (2009) Risk management: the importance of knowledge, *British Journal of Healthcare Assistants*, 3(7): 338–40.

Hally, H. (1999) Inquiries into the care of mentally ill people: the lessons, in T. Ryan (ed.) *Managing Crisis and Risk in Mental Health Nursing*. Cheltenham: Nelson Thornes.

Hamm, R.M. (1988) Clinical intuition and clinical analysis: expertise and the cognitive continuum, in J. Dowie and A. Elstein (eds) *Professional Judgement: A Reader in Clinical Decision Making*. Cambridge: Cambridge University Press.

Harrison, A. (2003) A guide to risk assessment, *Nursing Times*, 99(9): 44–5.

Hart, S., Kropp, P.R., Laws, D.R., Klaver, J., Logan, C. and Watt, K.A. (2003) *The Risk for Sexual Violence Protocol (RSVP): Structured Professional Guidelines for Assessing Risk of Sexual Violence*. Vancouver: The Institute Against Family Violence.

Ilgen, M.A., Czyz, E.K., Welsh, D.E., Zeber, J.E., Bauer, M.S. and Kilbourne, A.M. (2009) A collaborative therapeutic relationship and risk of suicidal ideation in patients with bipolar disorder, *Journal of Affective Disorders*, 115: 246–51.

Kaliniecka, H. and Shawe-Taylor, M. (2008) Promoting positive risk management: evaluation of a risk management panel, *Journal of Psychiatric and Mental Health Nursing*, 15: 654–61.

Kemshall, H. (2002) *Risk, Social Policy and Welfare*. Buckingham: Open University Press.

Kropp, P.R., Hart, S.D., Webster, C.D. and Eaves, D. (1995) *Manual for the Spousal Assault Risk Assessment Guide*, 2nd edn. Vancouver: British Columbia Institute on Family Violence.

Lamond, D. and Thompson, K. (2000) Intuition and analysis in decision making and choice, *Journal of Nursing Scholarship*, 4: 411–14.

Langan, J. and Lindow, V. (2004) *Living with Risk: Mental Health Service User Involvement in Risk Assessment and Management*. Bristol: Policy Press.

Martin, D. (2006). How to use non-verbal signs in assessments of suicide risk, *Nursing Times*, 102(2): 36–9.

McDonnell, A. and Gallon, I. (2006) Issues and concerns about control and restraint training: moving the debate forward, in J.R. Cutcliffe and M.F. Ward (eds) *Key Debates in Psychiatric/Mental Health Nursing*. Oxford: Churchill Livingstone.

McLean, J., Maxwell, M., Platt, S., Harris, F. and Jepson, R. (2008) *Risk and Protective Factors for Suicide and Suicidal Behaviour: A Literature Review*. Edinburgh: Scottish Government Social Research.

Mental Capacity Act (2005) *Mental Capacity Act Code of Practice Mental Capacity Act*. London: HMSO

Morgan, S. (2000) *Clinical Risk Management: A Clinical Tool and Practitioner Manual*. London: Sainsbury Centre for Mental Health.

National Institute for Clinical Excellence (NICE) (2004) *Self-harm: The Short-term Physical and Psychological Management and Secondary Prevention of Self-harm in Primary and Secondary Care*. London: National Institute for Clinical Excellence.

National Patient Safety Agency (NPSA) (2007) *Healthcare Risk Assessment Made Easy*. London: NPSA.

NHS Quality Improvement Scotland (2010) *Vital Systems, Supporting Healthcare Improvement in Scotland – Person-centred Safe and Effective Care: Clinical Governance and Risk Management a National Overview*. Edinburgh: NHS QIS.

NHS Scotland (2008) *The Art of Conversation: A Guide to Talking, Listening and Reducing Stigma Surrounding Suicide*. Edinburgh: NHS Scotland.

Nursing and Midwifery Council (NMC) (2010) *Standards for Pre-registration Nursing Education*. London: NMC.

Petch, E. (2001) Risk management in UK mental health services: an overvalued idea? *Psychiatric Bulletin*, 25: 203–5.

Pratt, D. (2001) Risk management in mental health, *Nursing Times*, 97(25): 37–8.

Ritchie, J.H., Dick, D. and Lingham, R. (1994) *Report of the Inquiry into the Care and Treatment of Christopher Clunis*. London: HMSO.

Roberts, G. and Holly, J. (1996) *Risk Management in Healthcare*. London: Witherby.

Ryan, T. (2000) Exploring the risk management strategies of mental health service users, *Health, Risk and Society*, 2(3): 267–82.

Scottish Executive (2000) *Report of the Committee on Serious Violent and Sexual Offenders*. London: HMSO.

Webster, C.D. and Hucker, S.J. (2007) Violence risk assessment and management, in A. Maden (ed.) *Treating Violence: A Guide to Risk Management in Mental Health*. Oxford: Oxford University Press.

Webster, C.D., Douglas, K.S., Eaves, D. and Hart, S.D. (1997) *HCR-20: Assessing Risk for Violence* (Version 2). Burnaby, BC: The Mental Health, Law, and Policy Institute of Simon Fraser University.

Webster, C.D., Nicholls, T.L., Martin, M.-L., Desmaris, M.A. and Brink (2006) Short Term Assessment of Risk and Treatability (START): the case for a new structured professional judgment scheme. *Behavioural Sciences and the Law*, 24: 747–66.

Wiseman, S. (2003). Brief intervention: reducing the repetition of deliberate self harm, *Nursing Times*, 99(35): 34–8.

Woods, P. and Kettles, A.M. (2009) Introduction, in P. Woods and A.M. Kettles (eds) *Risk Assessment and Management in Mental Health Nursing*. Oxford: Blackwell.

2 From communication skills to psychological interventions

Deborah Knott

Chapter aim and objectives

Aim

- To explore the importance of communication skills in the delivery of psychosocial interventions in mental health care.

Objectives

- To describe a range of communications skills used within the field of mental health care.
- To identify key aspects of communications skills that underpin the delivery of effective psychosocial interventions.
- To apply a range of communication skills to a scenario situation.

Introduction

> One cannot not communicate.
>
> (Watzlawick, 1967: 15)

> The single biggest problem in communication is the illusion that it has taken place.
>
> (George Bernard Shaw, 1913)

The aim of this chapter is to explore a range of communication skills that are integral to the delivery of effective psychosocial interventions in mental health care (Bowers, 2010). Mental health nurses conduct their interventions almost exclusively through communication and therefore the more effective the communication the more effective the intervention. It is important to consider that good communication alone is not sufficient to deliver a range of effective interventions, rather a therapeutic relationship and, within it, the interpersonal skills that build this relationship are the foundation on which effective interventions are built (O'Carroll and Park, 2007). The development of essential skills clusters for pre-registration nursing programmes acknowledge the crucial part communication skills play in the development of safe and competent practitioners by dedicating a whole section to care, compassion and communication.

The essence of care benchmarks for the fundamental aspects of care defines communication as: 'a process that involves a meaningful exchange between at least two

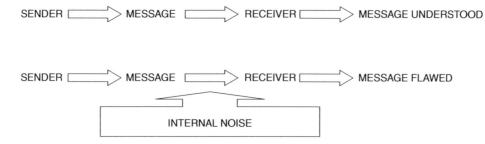

Figure 2.1 Sender/receiver communication model
Source: Shannon and Weaver (1949)

people to convey facts, needs, opinions, thoughts, feelings or other information through both verbal and non-verbal means, including face-to-face exchanges and the written word' (DoH, 2010: 7).

As previously mentioned the therapeutic relationship is the central component for safe and effective mental health practice (see also the introductory chapter). A purposeful and positive relationship is the means by which the nurse assists the service user in their journey to recovery (Rigby and Alexander, 2008). It is important that student nurses early on in their training develop the required relationship-building skills as ese will form the footbridge to their development as effective practitioners (O'Car and Park, 2007).

The sender/receiver model of communication is perhaps the best-known communication model and the simplest to understand. The process of communication begins with a sender, a message and a receiver. However, purposeful communication occurs only when the receiver has received the message *and* understood its purpose. A fairly simple transaction one would think. However, there are many factors to this process which could be incomplete or faulty. Many communications are subject to interference or 'internal noise' thus a problem with the transition develops because this 'noise' interferes with the successful completion of the process. Figure 2.1 is a simplistic representation of this process.

The internal noise can be from the sender, the receiver or affecting both parties in the process, and is usually as a result of inattention or distraction from an internal agenda. Consider the following scenario.

SCENARIO

Susan is a 19-year-old young woman who has been experiencing low mood for some time. Julie, the student nurse, has visited her in her home along with her mentor and has been asked to conduct a brief assessment of Susan's mental state. Julie is nervous

(continued)

as this is the first time she has been asked to do this alone. She begins the assessment well but is very conscious of her mentor watching, she stutters a little and struggles to ask Susan the questions on her prompt sheet. Susan has a good relationship with Julie's mentor and is resentful of the student's presence. Because of her feelings, Susan is monosyllabic, which serves to make Julie more hesitant.

Consider the possible presence of internal noise from:

1 Julie's point of view
2 Susan's point of view.

1 Julie's internal noise includes self-consciousness and nervousness at the fact she is being assessed. The prompt sheet may also be considered to be a distracting factor. Julie may also be conscious of Susan's monosyllabic answers and attempt to 'fill in the gaps'.
2 Susan's internal noise includes her low mood, she may be reluctant to give information to a student who is a stranger. Her resentment may mean she is unlikely to give out much information about her feelings.

Note: when working within the mental health setting, students should consider the presence of voices as possible internal noise affecting the channels of communication.

The development of skilled interpersonal communication has been evc ving for many years, with much of the positive evidence coming from the fields of counselling and psychotherapy. Studies examining service user perspectives on nurses' communication skills are rare. A study by McCabe (2004) looked at service users' opinions on nurse–patient communication and found that constantly the complaint was that nurses were too task orientated. An additional study by Chant et al. (2002) found that many student nurses were of the opinion that talking was not part of working and they felt the need to always look busy.

There is a wealth of evidence documenting the development of communication and interpersonal skills in the field of nursing, much of which has served to refocus the approach to mental health nursing from 'doing to' the service user to 'doing with' the service user (Brown et al., 2006). This collaborative approach necessitated an improvement in communication skills and the development of a focus on creating and sustaining the therapeutic relationship. The concept of effective communication being grounded in self-awareness was developed around this time (Burnard, 1996) and nurses were encouraged to examine how their knowledge and use of self affected their ability to communicate with service users and their carers. Brown et al. (2006) examined a wealth of evidence leading to recommendations about how best to train individuals to develop communication skills for use in the health-care setting.

Key issues identified by Brown et al. were:

• A multi-model approach adapted to individual situations is potentially the most effective way of developing interpersonal skills.
• Nurses should adopt use of self, and non-judgemental approaches.

- Experiential learning is the most effective way to develop skills.
- Contextual issues affect the way in which mental health nurses communicate.
- Clinically focused empathy enables the development of effective interpersonal skills.

Verbal communication

Verbal communication contains three major elements:

1 the words which are said by the sender, known as *vocals*
2 the way in which the sender says them, *paralanguage*
3 the way in which they are perceived by the receiver, called *metacommunication*.

Words are symbols used by people to classify and order information in ways that can be understood by themselves and others. The most important things to remember when communicating professionally are:

Cultural implications: not only ethnic, geographical or religious implications but also specific groups; for example, when you enter nursing you learn a new language and new set of connotations, this can make you feel overwhelmed and confused, a similar feeling to those entering a new culture with limited understanding.

Slang and jargon: different age groups in the same culture can attach different meanings to the same terms.

Consider possible responses in this next scenario.

SCENARIO

It is Julie's first day on an acute care in-patient unit. Just as she is leaving the office after a handover she is approach by Susan, who she met on her last placement, who is very distressed. Susan expresses relief to see a friendly face and demands that Julie take her home. Julie is unsure of how to respond to this as it is clear that Susan is in need of help. Julie wants to reassure Susan and relieve her distress but has no idea of how to respond as she has never dealt with this level of distress before.

1 How should Julie respond?
2 Consider what words Julie could use.
3 Consider how she says the words (tone, pitch).
4 What are the implications of her response?
5 Are there any specific aspects of verbal communication important for working with service users with depression?

1   Julie needs to ensure that she is able to reassure Susan and relieve her distress as far as possible in the first instance. She needs to take Susan somewhere private and sit her down, and ensure she is able to give her her full attention.

2   Julie should acknowledge Susan's distress – for example, 'I can see you are upset Susan, let's find somewhere to sit for a chat' – using words of encouragement showing she is available to listen to Susan's problems.

3   Speaking in a quiet tone, and keeping her voice level and steady, Julie should ask open questions inviting Susan to expand on her feelings.

4   Julie's response to Susan's distress is crucial; she needs to ensure she develops a level of trust in order to get Susan to open up her discussion. An insensitive or too probing a response could lead Susan to close down the discussion, restricting the flow of information.

5   Service users with depression are often reluctant to communicate, leaving the nurse with the difficult task of encouraging the service user to discuss their problems. Patience is crucial and the use of open questions points the service user towards giving longer answers which can then lead to further questioning by the nurse, based on the information received.

Non-verbal communication

As much as 60 to 65 per cent of the communication we use is non-verbal communication (Foley and Gentile, 2010). Our body language is often the way that we truly communicate when the words we are saying are insufficient (Chambers, 2003). Angry people can, without any words, convey their anger: their stance, proximity, facial expression and gestures leave us in no doubt as to how they are feeling. Depressed individuals often convey their mood by the way they are sitting, their eye contact or their withdrawal from the environment around them.

There are a myriad of different types of body language.

Facial expressions: can hide or show your feelings. Nurses must be acutely aware of their facial expression when interacting with service users, being careful not to convey negative feelings, but showing interest and openness.

Eye contact: is crucial in communication. We look more at people we like and a higher degree of eye contact often conveys a close relationship. We use eye contact to catch a person's attention and to initially engage. Appropriate eye contact can instantly create a connection and indicate interest between the service user and the nurse. Conversely, prolonged eye contact (staring) could indicate hostility.

Gestures: replace or illustrate speech, they are often used to release tension and can indicate aggression or defeat, or can be encouraging.

Posture: can be said to be one of the most important things to consider when approaching a service user. A closed posture is unlikely to invite conversations, whereas an open posture can indicate willingness to engage in discussion.

Head nods: convey agreement or acknowledgement of what is being said.

Orientation: the angle you are to another person can make communication easy or difficult, particularly with those who may be hard of hearing or whose vision is impaired. Standing or sitting directly opposite the service user or at a very slight angle can show openness and willingness to engage in conversation.

Proximity: people have different comfort levels.

Touch: should be used with *caution*, some people's personal boundaries are much further than others. It can be comforting, but it can also be misinterpreted.

Appearance: people perceive you differently depending on the type of clothes you wear – for example, police officer uniform = authority.

When the actual words are not making sense, body language can give you the clues you need to adapt your communication appropriately to the situation. However, non-verbal cues cannot be interpreted in a vacuum: the context of the communication needs to be taken into account. Hand gestures can mean one thing in one country and an entirely different thing in another!

Consider the non-verbal communication in this scenario.

SCENARIO

Upon beginning a late shift Julie spots Susan sitting in a corner with her head in her hands. She is uncommunicative and does not respond to Julie's attempts to discover the problem. When Julie asks her what is wrong she turns away and refuses to make eye contact.

1   What do you conclude about Julie's mood from her non-verbal behaviour?
2   How would you respond to the situation?
3   Consider your body language; what should you be aware of when approaching Susan?

1   Susan's body language is closed and defensive: she physically turns away when approached, clearly showing reluctance to engage in any communication. This could indicate extreme distress, low mood, or even anger. Her refusal to make eye contact could indicate that she is embarrassed or that she is determined not to engage in any communication with Julie.
2   Julie should acknowledge Susan's distress and be patient. She should tell Susan that she is willing to listen when she is ready to talk, and take a seat next to her. She should avoid asking Susan what the problem is after the initial questioning and should consider 'Is there anything I could do to help?'
3   Julie should be aware of Susan's closed body language and ensure that her own is open, indicating that she is approachable and willing to engage in conversation. She should ensure she sits where Susan can see her, remembering not to invade Susan's personal space.

Active listening is a way of listening to someone involving more than just an 'open ear'. It involves a two-way process that improves the process of communication but ensuring the listener hears what is being said as well as what is not being said (non-verbal cues) (Kacperek, 1997; Shipley, 2010). It is a structured form of listening which relies on the listener being able to convey understanding of what the speaker is saying, and is much more than the factual recording of the words. This is done by a series of techniques including responding appropriately, summarizing and reflecting back what is said to check understanding.

Several things need to be taken into account when employing active listening skills (Chambers, 2003; Bowers, 2010). The setting is important: it should, where possible, be chosen with care to avoid interruptions or excess noise and distraction. The listener should be aware that listening with care and attention is a caring response and as such requires perceptions through several senses. The listener needs to constantly check their existing knowledge about the situation against new information. Active listening requires the listener to give up any preconceptions about the person held prior to the session and listen with an open mind, which should be reflected throughout their body language. During active listening periods one should use non-verbal cues to show attention, nodding or acknowledging with an 'mm' or 'aha' tells the person that you are attentive to their information and are understanding what they are saying. Posture, eye contact, position, gestures and distance from the service user all carry messages about the listener's degree of interest and attention.

Reflecting back what has just been heard may initially seem strange but gives clear feedback that what has been said has been received and understood. Reflecting content back to the service user lets them know that any implied message (often about feelings) which has not been expressed directly has also been understood.

Alongside listening skills it is appropriate to consider the use of silence in thera-peutic communication (Kacperek, 1997; Shipley, 2010). Many people are wary of using silence and feel uncomfortable with a period of silence in conversation; however, in mental health nursing this is an important technique. Periods of silence allow the ser-vice user to consider what information they wish to convey, and allow the listener to consider the information provided and the most appropriate response to the service user. Comfortableness with silence is often a good indicator of listening skill, that the worker is at ease and able to contain their own anxieties in order to concentrate on the service user and allow them 'thinking time'.

This chapter has considered so far how to negotiate verbal and non-verbal methods of communication and how to listen actively to what is being communicated but, as stated earlier, communication is a two-way process so there needs to be a response on the part of the listener. There are several ways to respond and expand conversation, one of which is asking questions to elicit further information. However one needs to consider how the question is framed in order to gain the most information.

Asking open questions can help the service user to explore their experience them-selves with minimal prompting. 'Can you say a little more about how you felt when . . .?' opens up discussion and allows the service user to actually think about their feelings in the situation. A closed question – for example, 'Did you feel angry when . . . .?' – suggests a one-word answer 'Yes', immediately closing down the discussion and not inviting any further exploration of feelings. This is less exploratory and potentially less helpful to the service user.

The self

In order to work within the therapeutic relationship it is essential that the student nurse develop empathy skills (Jack and Smith, 2007). These skills allow the mental health worker to recognize and acknowledge the experiences and feelings of a service user without having actually experienced themselves what the service user is experiencing.

The concept was first described in 1887 by Lipps, a German psychologist, as 'being able to fully understand the experience of another without loss of self' (Arnold and Boggs, 2003: 120). In other words, being able to identify with the service user's thoughts and feelings without giving too much of yourself, that is, self-disclosure.

Empathic skills include the employment of active listening, as described earlier in this chapter, and genuine interest in the service user as a person rather than an illness (Shipley, 2010). Acceptance of the service user, coupled with a caring, compassionate attitude and a range of interpersonal skills, particularly non-verbal skills including the use of eye contact, help to develop an empathic approach to client care.

The employment of a clinically focused empathic approach in mental health nursing in particular is not always easy. By the very nature of the illness, service users often hide what they are really feeling, through fear of being ridiculed or dismissed, or perhaps they are fearful of being detained in hospital or discharged too soon (Bowers, 2010). The mental health nurse needs to be aware of these issues and take into account the service user's non-verbal cues as well as their verbal answers. Often the real emotions lie behind what is not being said rather than what is being said.

Getting the empathic response right, by conveying genuine interest, acceptance and caring, is likely to assist the mental health worker in creating a secure emotional bond with the service user, creating a safe, trustworthy clinical environment within which the service user can develop and expand coping strategies, reduce stress and improve their mental health.

Consider your response in this scenario.

SCENARIO

You are spending some time with Susan who has been discharged and is now under the care of the Community Mental Health Team. She discloses during the session that her uncle who sexually abused her from an early age has just died. She begins to describe the experience and says she feels guilty and angry but also is sorry he is dead.

1　Think about your facial expression, how, non-verbally could you convey empathy?
2　What would you need to consider before responding verbally?
3　What emotions do you need to convey?

1   Julie should keep her facial expression neutral and interested. It is crucial that no horror or disgust is conveyed in case Susan misinterprets the expression to be directed at her. An open posture, leaning slightly forward should be adopted. Eye contact should be considered, not too direct or staring.

2   Julie needs to consider her own feelings about the situation and that her response may influence the rest of Susan's disclosure. Julie needs to measure her response carefully to avoid alienating Susan.

3   Julie needs to ensure that she conveys acceptance and positive regard, while encouraging further communication.

Self-awareness is a crucial element of interpersonal skills and the higher the individual's level of self-awareness the more likely it is to produce a safe practitioner; and a high level of self-awareness is a critical ingredient of the nurse–patient relationship. The 'self' is a complex concept, not easily defined or agreed upon. Each theorist has his/her own definition for that part of us that is concerned with thinking, feeling, valuing, evaluating and so forth.

Two examples are detailed here; however, there are many and varied definitions available: 'Whilst, in one sense, the mind and body are one, in another, they are different if only that the mind is a thing, an object of the world, whilst the "self" is a construct' (Burnard, 2002: 632); 'The means by which a person gains knowledge and understanding of all aspects of self-concept . . . the nurse's self-concept is as important as that of the clients . . . self-awareness provides an inner frame of reference for connecting with the experiences of others' (Arnold and Boggs, 2003: 109).

The common thread in all definitions of self is the idea that there are two elements of ourselves: the outer, public experience which includes movement, speech, eye contact, touch, proximity to others, gestures and facial expressions; conversely, there is also the inner, private experience, which includes thinking, feeling, sensing and intuiting. These two elements work together in order to produce the essential elements of each individual. The nurse must strive to increase their self-awareness in order to develop into an effective practitioner who can build and sustain safe, therapeutic relationships with service users, their families and within their working relationships (DoH, 2006b).

Appropriate self-disclosure is a tool used in order to build up a therapeutic relationship. Often, self-disclosure is reciprocal and the sharing of information between two people increases the bond, builds trust and allows the service user to feel empathy from the nurse (Hargie, 2006).

It is important to remember professional boundaries when disclosing to clients/patients. The information disclosed may involve information about your values and beliefs, or your wishes, or be about self qualities or characteristics. The nurse–patient relationship is a continually developing characteristic and the exchange of information over a period of time helps to build and solidify the relationship to the point where it needs to be dissolved and closed (Bach and Grant, 2009).

Caution is always necessary when considering disclosing information to service users. Ask yourself the following:

1   Why are you telling them the information?

2   How will this information affect the therapeutic relationship?

3   How will this information affect your ability to do your job with that person?

4   What would be the positives of this disclosure?
5   What might be the negatives of this disclosure?

One way to safeguard your practice and develop your skills and knowledge is to become an effective reflective practitioner (see also the introductory chapter) (Jack and Smith, 2007). The process of reflection is a simple one, but one that many nurses find difficult to employ. Rolfe defines reflection as:

> Reflection is a process of thinking, feeling, imagining, and learning by considering what has happened in the past, what might have happened if things had been done differently, what is currently happening, and what could possibly happen in the future. Reflection might in some cases be a dispassionate and objective review of the facts of the matter, or it might focus predominately on the feelings and personal reactions of the person who is reflecting or of someone else involved in the situation.
>
> (Rolfe, 2011: 12)

The crucial element of reflection is that it needs to be a cyclical process; nurses need to reflect on the incident, make sense of it, then action-plan for the future (Rolfe, 2011). This action plan is the means by which nurses' learning from experience is put into practice and further develops their skills.

Driscoll's model of reflection (Ooijen, 2003) is thought to be the simplest model to follow:

1   *What?* An event or experience from clinical practice is described after which some elements are selected for further reflection.
2   *So what?* The event is analysed and any learning from this is made conscious.
3   *Now what?* Action is planned and carried out.

Nurses need to familiarize themselves with their preferred model of reflection and utilize it throughout their career in order to improve practice, support learning, respond imaginatively to any complex situations and challenge 'common-sense assumptions' that traditionally inform actions. This will help nurses to develop themselves as individuals, and their practice as a whole, while maintaining a safe environment for themselves and the service user.

Consider your response in this scenario.

SCENARIO

You are visiting Susan who has improved greatly since her discharge from hospital. She tells you that she sees you as a friend and doesn't feel like you are a nurse at all. As she is around your age she asks if you would like to meet up one evening to go for a night on the town. You agree that this may be fun and vaguely arrange to set a date at the end of the month. When leaving the visit you feel a little uneasy.

Reflect on the situation using Driscoll's model.

Have you made the right decision?
How did the situation make you feel?
How will you conduct the next visit to Susan?
What do you need to do in order to resolve your conflict?

Communication skills and psychological interventions

The effective communicator is agreed by many to be a safe practitioner. A range of good, effective communication skills is the foundation for a safe nurse–service user relationship within which elements such as trust and openness allow for effective, collaborative risk taking and risk management (see also Chapter 1) (Doyle et al., 2007; Jack and Smith, 2007; O'Carroll and Park, 2007; Boscart, 2009). Being safe underpins all interactions within the nurse–patient relationship. The Nursing and Midwifery Council (NMC) has considered this and provided guidance to all nurses of safe professional conduct (see also Chapter 11): 'As a professional, you are personally accountable for actions and omissions in your practice, and must always be able to justify your decision' (NMC, 2008: 2).

Nurses have a duty of care at all times to the people in their care, and effective interpersonal and communication skills allow the nurse to interpret messages accurately and ensure all parties understand the situation before acting appropriately to minimize risk and ensure safe practice (Doyle et al., 2007; Jack and Smith, 2007; Bowers, 2010). Individual trusts have Safeguarding of Vulnerable Adults policy documentation which ensures that nurses take safe practice seriously. Guidelines also assist the mental health worker in their roles and responsibilities in keeping both service users and workers as safe as possible, in what is often an unpredictable environment (DoH, 2006a).

The Department of Health document *Best Practice Competencies and Capabilities for Pre-registration Mental Health Nurses in England* and *The Chief Nursing Officer's Review of Mental Health Nursing* (2006b) give guidance for standards to be achieved specifically by student nurses prior to registration. Among these detailed competencies is recognition of the student nurses' responsibility to develop themselves to become responsible practitioners at the point of registration (DoH, 2006a: 5). Alongside these documents, the new *Essence of Care 2010, Benchmarks for the Fundamental Aspects of Care* (DoH, 2010) has a section on good communication skills, detailing how the safe practitioner develops their interpersonal and communication skills and interaction with service users, carers, other professionals and members of the public.

A study by Bowers (2010) conducted a survey of expert nurses and the skills they used to communicate with service users. The conclusions drawn from the research suggest that the communication techniques reported in this study should be applied to all nurse–service user interactions throughout mental health service provision. The study proposes that developing skills in this area would enhance collaboration and cooperation between the service user and their mental health worker, thus increasing service-user satisfaction with the care they receive.

Taking this into consideration, it is with a good grounding in effective communication that the student nurse is then able to develop a range of psychological interventions designed to meet the needs of service users with a wide range of mental health problems (DoH, 2006b; O'Carroll and Park, 2007; Doyle et al., 2007; Boscart, 2009; NMC, 2010).

Summary of the key points

Effective psychological interventions are based on effective communication skills which should be framed within the therapeutic relationship.

Communication consists of a 'sender', a 'receiver' and a message. The message can be distorted or misinterpreted by the presence of internal noise. Active listening encourages disclosure and the development of the process of two-way communication.

Communication can be divided into verbal communication and non-verbal communication.

Nurses need to develop good self-awareness in order to be empathic communicators. A good level of self-awareness enables the nurse to maintain safe practice. Nurses should also develop themselves as reflective practitioners in order to expand their knowledge and skills.

Quick quiz

1　Give a definition of communication.
2　Describe a model of communication.
3　Name two aspects of verbal communication.
4　Name two ways in which we communicate non-verbally.
5　What is the likely outcome of asking an open question rather than a closed one?
6　Give two examples of an open question/closed question.
7　What is 'the self' and why is self-awareness so important in nursing?
8　Outline a model of reflection.
9　Why is the ability to reflect on one's practice so important in nursing?
10　What does the Nursing and Midwifery Council say about communication?

References

Arnold, A. and Boggs, K. (2003) *Interpersonal Relationships: Professional Communication Skills for Nurses*. St Louis, MO: Elsevier Science.

Bach, S. and Grant, A. (2009) *Communication and Interpersonal Skills for Nurses*. Exeter: Learning Matters.

Boscart, V.M. (2009) A communication intervention for nursing staff in chronic care, *Journal of Advanced Nursing*, 65(9): 1823–32.

Bowers, L. (2010) How expert nurses communicate with acutely psychotic patients, *Mental Health Practice*, 13(7): 24–26.

Brown, B., Crawford, P. and Carter, R. (2006) *Evidence Based Health Communication*. Maidenhead: Open University Press.

Burnard, P. (1996) *Acquiring Interpersonal Skills: A Handbook of Experiential Learning for Health Care Professionals*. London: Chapman and Hall.

Burnard, P. (2002) Book review: Evidence based counselling and psychological therapies: research and applications, *Journal of Psychiatric and Mental Health Nursing*, 9(5): 632.

Chambers, S. (2003) Use of non-verbal-communication to improve nursing care, *British Journal of Nursing*, 12(14): 874–8.

Chant, S., Jenkinson, T., Randle, J. and Russell, G. (2002) Communication skills: some problems in nursing education and practice, *Journal of Clinical Nursing*, 11: 12–21.

Department of Health (2006a) *From Values to Action: The Chief Nursing Officer's Review of Mental Health Nursing*. London: Department of Health.

Department of Health (2006b) *Best Practice Competencies and Capabilities for Pre-registration Mental Health Nurses in England: The Chief Nursing Officer's Review of Mental Health Nursing*. London: Department of Health.

Department of Health (2010) *Essence of Care 2010: Benchmarks for the Fundamental Aspects of Care*. London: Department of Health.

Doyle, L., Keogh, B. and Morrissey, J. (2007) Caring for patients with suicidal behaviour: an exploratory study, *British Journal of Nursing*, 16(19): 1218–22.

Foley, G. and Gentile, J. (2010) Non verbal communication in psychotherapy, *Psychiatry*, 7(6): 38–44.

Hargie, O. (2006) *The Handbook of Communication Skills*. Hove: Routledge.

Jack, K. and Smith, A. (2007) Promoting self-awareness in nurses to improve nursing practice, *Nursing Standard*, 21(32): 47–52.

Kacperek, L. (1997) Non-verbal communication: the importance of listening, *British Journal of Nursing*, 6(5): 275–9.

McCabe, C. (2004) Nurse patient communication: an exploration of patients' experiences, *Journal of Clinical Nursing*, 13: 41–9.

Nursing and Midwifery Council (NMC) (2008) *The Code: Standards of Conduct, Performance and Ethics for Nurses and Midwives*. London: Nursing and Midwifery Council.

Nursing and Midwifery Council (NMC) (2010) *Standards for Pre-registration Nursing Education*. London: Nursing and Midwifery Council.

O'Carroll, M. and Park, A. (2007) *Essential Mental Health Nursing Skills*. London: Mosby.

Ooijen, E.V. (2003) *Clinical Supervision Made Easy: The 3 Step Method*. Edinburgh: Elsevier.

Rigby, P. and Alexander, J. (2008) Building positive therapeutic relationships, in J. Dooher (ed.) *Fundamental Aspects of Mental Health Nursing*. London: Quay Books.

Rolfe, G. (2011) Knowledge and practice, in G. Rolfe, M. Jasper and D. Freshwater (eds) *Critical Reflection in Practice: Generating Knowledge for Care*, 2nd edn. Basingstoke: Palgrave Macmillan.

Shannon, C.E. and Weaver, W. (1949) *A Mathematical Model of Communication*. Urbana, IL: University of Illinois Press.

Shipley, S.D. (2010) Listening: a concept analysis, *Nursing Forum*, 45(2): 125–34.

Watzlawick, P., Beavin, J.H. and Jackson, D.D. (1967) *Pragmatics of Human Communication*. New York: W.W. Norton.

3 Psychological interventions in psychosis

Ged Carney and Grahame Smith

Chapter aim and objectives

Aim

- To explore the conceptual basis of the term psychosis and its relationship to caregiving within the field of mental health.

Objectives

- To identify psychosis in terms of theories, approaches and classification.
- To describe and critique the evidence base underpinning the care of individuals with a psychosis.
- To describe, analyse and apply psychological interventions to the care of individuals with a psychosis.

What is a psychosis?

The first part of this chapter will explore psychosis in terms of its location within the mental disorders, looking more in depth at the main psychotic disorder: schizophrenia (Davey, 2008). The second part of the chapter will look at the evidence base for the treatment of schizophrenia, and the third part of the chapter will explore the application of psychological interventions within a scenario. At this juncture it is also important to recognize that any psychological interventions need to take into account the point articulated in Chapter 1, that any subsequent psychological interventions need to be grounded in the mental health service user's narrative (Merleau-Ponty, [1945]1962; Bracken and Thomas, 2005; Hamilton and Roper, 2006).

As a useful starting point Davey provides the following definition of psychosis and its symptoms:

> Psychotic symptoms can be crippling and are characterized by disturbances in thought and language, sensory perception, emotional regulation and behaviour. Sufferers may experience sensory hallucinations and also develop thought disorders which may lead to pervasive false beliefs or delusions about themselves and the world around them. Individuals with psychotic symptoms may often withdraw from normal social interaction because of these disturbances of perception and thought, and this can result in poor educational

performance, increasing unproductivity, difficulties in interpersonal relationships, neglect of day-to-day activities and a preoccupation with a personal
world to the exclusion of others.

(Davey, 2008: 207)

It has to be remembered that the type of definition above is framed through the lens
of a number of conceptual models only some of which are psychological. The medical
model also plays a part; not everyone will agree with this type of definition, so feel
free to look at other definitions (Bracken and Thomas, 2005; Department of Health,
2006a; 2006b).

Psychosis is also viewed as occurring within a number of mental disorders, such
as schizophrenia, schizophreniform disorder and schizoaffective disorder, bipolar disorder and major depressive disorder, to name a few (Van Os and Kapur, 2009; Barrett
et al., 2010). In terms of symptomology, psychosis, according to Van Os and Kapur
(2009), can broadly be clustered into four symptom categories: delusions and hallucinations; lack of motivation and social withdrawal; memory and attention difficulties;
and difficulty in regulating mood.

Bak et al. (2003: 349) make the point that 'not all individuals who experience
psychotic symptoms develop a need for care'. What is important is how the individual
interacts with their psychotic experience; where an individual experiencing psychotic
symptoms is able to socially function, such as work and/or maintain good social contact, the less likely is their need for care (Bak et al., 2003). Where care is required, early
intervention can be crucial, particularly the quality and effectiveness of the care given
(Addington and Gleeson, 2005; Bird et al., 2010).

Traditionally schizophrenia, in which personal, social and occupational functioning can significantly deteriorate, is seen as the main psychotic disorder and as with all
mental disorders it is currently diagnosed via the *Diagnostic and Statistical Manual of
Mental Disorders IV* (DSM-IV TR) and the 10th International Classification of Diseases
(ICD-10) (Comer, 2008; Davey, 2008; Van Os and Kapur, 2009; Akal and Dogan, 2010).
Schizophrenia as a clinical label originated from the work of Kraepelin who, in 1887,
described schizophrenia as dementia praecox. Kraepelin believed that the condition
was an early form of dementia. It was Bleuler, in 1911, moving away from the idea
of an early form of dementia, who coined the term schizophrenia: 'schiz' meaning
'split' and 'phren' meaning 'mind' (Davey, 2008; Gillam and Williams, 2008). In a
contemporary context Van Os and Kapur highlight that:

A debate exists as to whether the term schizophrenia, which refers to a state of
so-called split mind, should be retained in DSM-V and ICD-11. Japan was the
first country to abandon the term schizophrenia, and modified the name of
the illness from Seishin Bunretsu Byo (mind-split disease) into Togo Shitcho
Sho (integration-dysregulation syndrome). The change of name had an instant
response. Most psychiatrists started using it in the first year, bringing about
an improved communication of diagnosis to patients and better perception of
the disorder. Thus, the term schizophrenia will continue to evolve; however,
the underlying mechanisms and the effect on the person will not change.

(Van Os and Kapur, 2009: 636)

Around 1 per cent of the population in the UK have a diagnosis of schizophrenia, which according to Berry and Haddock (2008: 420) equates to '210,000 people with the diagnosis at any one time'. Schizophrenia affects people in different ways but generally there are positive symptoms (distortions of normal functioning), such as hallucinations, delusions and thought disorder, and negative symptoms (loss of normal functions), such as lack of volition, poverty of thought and poverty of speech (Burton, 2006; Berry and Haddock, 2008; Davey, 2008; Gillam and Williams, 2008). Symptoms can persist over a long duration where individuals may experience frequent relapses even when taking antipsychotic medication (Berry and Haddock, 2008; Gillam and Williams, 2008).

Schizophrenia is further divided into sub-types: disorganised, previously known as Hebephrenia; Catatonic; Paranoid; and Residual (Comer, 2008; Davey, 2008). Generally schizophrenia is diagnosed (see DSM IV-TR for greater detail) if at least two of the following symptoms are present for a significant portion of time within a period of one month:

- Hallucinations
- Delusions
- Disorganised speech
- Catatonic behaviour
- Disorganised behaviour
- Negative symptoms

(Sadock and Sadock, 2010: 146)

The cause of schizophrenia is not clear but there are a number of risk factors which relate to an individual developing the condition, such as presence among first-degree relatives, age, gender, prenatal poor nutrition, obstetric complications and low social class (Davey, 2008; Akal and Dogan, 2010).

To summarize this section, the following scenario provides an illustrative example within the mental health-care field of the general impact a psychosis can have upon the individual; we will look at this scenario in more detail in the psychological interventions section.

SCENARIO

Paul is a 22-year-old man living at home with his mum, dad and older sister. He was taken by his mother to the local crisis team following an individual appointment with her GP who was the family's GP. On arrival his mum stated that she can no longer cope with her son who has withdrawn to his room in the house and does not interact with other members of his family. It has come to breaking point as she has only just found out that he dropped out of college six months ago.

On interview with Paul he describes how he has been hearing voices which constantly put him down. This has led to him withdrawing from his friends and he reports that he feels down and suicidal. It is ascertained that Paul has no plan or intent to act on his feelings of suicide.

Evidence-based practice

As previously mentioned early detection and early intervention are important in the treatment of a psychosis and also just as important in the treatment of schizophrenia (International Early Psychosis Writing Group, 2005). Gillam and Williams (2008: 84) make the point that: 'Early detection is important given that patients who present with a very acute and sudden onset illness (with prominent positive symptoms) tend to have a better prognosis following treatment than those with a more insidious onset.' Further, in relation to the importance of early intervention and managing risk via an early intervention team Ashir and Marlowe (2009: 226) highlight: 'The importance in early intervention team is emphasised due to the increased risk of violence, vulnerability and of suicide for those with a diagnosis of schizophrenia.'

Even though an early intervention team will focus on mental health service users who have an increased risk, it does not necessarily mean that risky behaviour is an inherent part of schizophrenia; each case has to be risk-assessed on a case-by-case basis (Ashir and Marlowe, 2009; Eales, 2009). That said, Barrett et al. (2010) highlight that early intervention within the early onset of a psychotic presentation does appear generally to have a positive effect on reducing risky behaviour, in this case suicidal behaviour.

A central concern about delivering the right level of service whether it is early intervention or wider health and social care is that not all individuals with a diagnosis of schizophrenia are accessing the appropriate type of service. This may in part be due to such issues as inadequate mental health resources and/or individuals with mental health needs being socially excluded (Berry and Haddock, 2008). Van Os and Kapur make the point that:

> Schizophrenia does not just affect mental health; patients with a diagnosis of schizophrenia die 12–15 years before the average population, with this mortality difference increasing in recent decades. Thus, schizophrenia causes more loss of lives than do most cancers and physical illnesses. Although some deaths are suicides, the main reason for increased mortality is related to physical causes, resulting from decreased access to medical care and increased frequency of routine risk factors (poor diet, little exercise, obesity, and smoking).
>
> (Van Os and Kapur, 2009: 635)

One way these issues have been addressed is through the development of core treatment guidelines such as the guidance published by the National Institute for Health and Clinical Excellence (NICE), which was first published in 2002 and updated in 2009 (Berry and Haddock, 2008; Gillam and Williams, 2008; NICE, 2009; Prytys et al., 2011). In terms of psychological interventions Prytys et al. provide the following useful summary which should be read in conjunction with the full NICE guidance:

> In 2002, the National Institute for Clinical Excellence (NICE) published its first clinical guideline, providing evidence-based recommendations for the care and treatment of adults with schizophrenia. The NICE guideline was produced on the basis of an extensive review of evidence for psychological treatments for schizophrenia (NICE, 2002) and contains 69 recommendations of which 14 are concerned with psychological interventions (Pilling and Price, 2006). Family intervention (FI) and cognitive–behavioural therapy (CBT) for psychosis are recommended as first-line treatments for those with a schizophrenia spectrum diagnosis and persisting positive symptoms or who are at risk of relapse (NICE, 2002). More recently, an updated version of the NICE guideline for schizophrenia (NICE, 2009) has been published which continues to recommend both CBT and FI for schizophrenia.
>
> (Prytys et al., 2011: 49)

Along with psychological interventions antipsychotic medication is also mentioned in the NICE guidance (NICE, 2009). According to Barber and Robertson (2009) antipsychotic medication is an important intervention, although Kuller et al. (2010) make the point that in terms of symptom control even second-generation antipsychotic medication is not sufficient as a treatment on its own.

Generally, antipsychotic medication can be divided into two groups: typical and atypical. Typical or first-generation antipsychotics were developed in the 1950s while atypical or second-generation antipsychotics have, in the main, been developed since the 1990s (Davey, 2008; Barber and Robertson, 2009). In terms of therapeutic action, typical antipsychotics block dopamine transmission mainly at dopamine receptor D2 sites within the brain, and are associated with more side effects than atypical antipsychotics, which include a variety of movement disorders (Barber and Robertson, 2009; Pandya, 2009). Atypical antipsychotics also block dopamine transmission but at dopamine receptor D1 and dopamine receptor D4 sites; side effects include weight gain, diabetes and, in some cases, blood disorders (Barber and Robertson, 2009). Owing to the potential physical health impact of antipsychotics it is important that prior to starting medication mental health service users undergo a baseline electrocardiogram (ECG) to exclude any cardiac problems (prolonged QT interval) (Pandya, 2009). While continuing on antipsychotic medication the mental health service user needs to be monitored for potential metabolic problems which may lead to an increase risk of cardiovascular disease and diabetes (Pandya, 2009).

As previously noted medication is not sufficient on its own. On this basis psychological therapies should also be offered; the psychological therapy that is specifically recommended in schizophrenia is cognitive behavioural therapy (Fung et al., 2008; Kuller et al., 2010). Even as a specific therapy a cognitive behavioural approach in the treatment of schizophrenia is not one size fits all, but it does have common features such as the establishment of a collaborative therapeutic relationship, identifying psychotic experiences within a dysfunctional to normality continuum, and focusing on reducing psychotic symptoms through modifying thought processes and enhancing coping strategies (Westbrook et al., 2007; Kuller et al., 2010).

Other psychological approaches or psychosocial treatments have been found to be beneficial, such as supported employment, family intervention and social skills training (Fung et al., 2008). These approaches are seen to be most beneficial in terms of preventing social isolation, promoting social functioning, relapse prevention and alleviating symptoms, especially negative symptoms.

The key challenges for the mental health nurse in utilizing the full range of psychosocial approaches are the need to develop the required level of skill and the need to maintain these skills through good supervision (DoH, 2006a; Berry and Haddock, 2008). As stated in Chapter 1, one of the key roles of the mental health nurse is to maintain, promote and ensure that the patient's narrative is at the core of any intervention base. This includes diagnosis, treatment and outcomes, and can be encapsulated within the recovery process. 'Researchers often define recovery as an extended period of remission from psychotic symptoms. Clinicians may define recovery as an improvement in global functioning and lastly for consumers recovery is a matter of retaining a meaningful life' (Torgalsboen and Rund, 2010: 71). Furthermore Deegan (1996: 93) stated: 'The goal of the recovery process is not to become normal. The goal is to embrace our human vocation of becoming more deeply, fully human. The goal is not normalisation. The goal is to become the unique awesome never to be repeated human being we are called to be.'

While the explanations above show there is no single universal definition of recovery, it can be said to have particular components: the service user's narrative (see Lovejoy, 1984; Frere, 2010); a fluidity of process (see Barker and Buchanan-Barker, 2005); and it is outcomes based (see Mackeith and Burns, 2008). Recovery is a move away from the historical medically based field of mental health to one that is seen as humanistic. Models of recovery include the 'strengths model' (Rapp and Goscha 2006), the 'tidal model' (Barker and Buchanan-Barker, 2005), which is particularly relevant for mental health nurses, and the 'wellness recovery action plan' (Copeland, 1997). These models create a framework and context within which the mental health nurse can provide psychological interventions to enable people to self-manage their mental health. Further key evidence can be found in a Department of Health publication, *New Horizons* (2009), which emphasizes the need to prevent mental ill health and promote well-being, indicating that the mental health nurse should take a holistic approach when working with people who have an experience of psychosis.

The role defined for the professional within recovery is seen as similar to one of a facilitator who utilizes their professionalism while learning from the expert, namely the service user, at the same time (Shepherd et al., 2008). Lester et al. (2005) identified that listening is highly valued by service users as a helpful part of the therapeutic alliance relationship (see also Chapter 2). The application of such therapeutic skills as active listening is also an important part in the process of facilitating the service user through their journey to recovery (Shepherd et al., 2008).

Psychological interventions and scenario

The chapter scenario continues.

SCENARIO

Immediate treatment options are discussed with Paul, including an in-patient stay. Paul stated that he would like to remain at home and a plan is drawn up for involvement from the early intervention team and a prescription for an atypical antipsychotic is completed. The assessment by the Early Intervention Team identified CBT, family education and allocation to the Assertive Outreach Team as initial interventions. The Assertive Outreach Team has an allotment aimed specifically at young men. This enabled Paul to develop his interpersonal skills and also practise some of the skills that had been identified in his CBT sessions with his nurse. Paul started on one hour per day and gradually built this up to a day a week. He also started to connect with his friends once again. As Paul was engaging more with people around him, he developed a wellness action recovery plan with his mental health nurse. This plan included a wellness box, the things that help, what doesn't help, trigger factors, early warning signs and a crisis plan. All through the process, outcomes were measured using the recovery star (Mackeith and Burns, 2008).

When offering CBT, the first stage, which can take some time, is to identify the areas the service user wants to work on first. This has to be led by the service user as it highlights the importance the service user puts on each individual aspect of living with a psychosis. In Paul's case he wanted to know about his condition and his medications. Over a short period of time Paul, working alongside the nurse, was encouraged to identify his personal perspective of psychosis while the education programme was being delivered. This enabled a therapeutic alliance to be formed and gave Paul the opportunity to explore what the diagnosis of schizophrenia meant to him.

In the initial stages of CBT Paul was facilitated to identify the negative effect of his psychosis, which for Paul was losing all his friends and becoming socially withdrawn. The nurse then enabled Paul to link his thoughts (*my friends will think I am mad*) with his actions (*not seeing his friends*) and his feelings (*sadness*). At this juncture Paul was supported to challenge his thought processes, while at the same time behavioural goals were set that focused on increasing his social functioning. As an outcome of this process Paul was then able to start attending a young men's group that was facilitated by the Early Intervention Team. It is useful to note that the NICE guidelines (2009) recommend that the mental health nurse should consider the use of a suitable instruction book when delivering CBT. Although no specific book is recommended by NICE, you might consider looking at *A Clinician's Guide to Mind Over Mood* by Pradesky and Greenberger (1995).

The nurse should aim to consult with the family and identify any knowledge deficits (Dixon and Lehman, 1995; International Early Psychosis Writing Group, 2005). In this case the family wanted to know what psychosis is, what medications are most useful and what are the side effects, how to help Paul (useful coping strategies) and what is the best treatment. As a result of this consultation process the nurse will need to formulate an education plan which will be delivered during a six-week time period.

An example of a training plan is given in Table 3.1.

Using the training plan the family were able to recognize some 'helpful and unhelpful' behaviours. An example of an unhelpful behaviour was family members checking on Paul by knocking on his door every hour on the hour. An example of a helpful behaviour was where mum and Paul had agreed to have one meal per day in the family kitchen.

To further support Paul a motivational interviewing approach was used; this approach was originally described by Miller (1983) and then refined by Miller and Rollnick (1991), and was first introduced as an intervention for people who had alcohol abuse (see Chapter 6 for further details). There is a growing trend of using this approach in the field of psychosis (Rusch and Corrigan, 2002) as it is considered to be client centred and semi-directive in its delivery. In a therapeutic setting, the interviewer when working with a service user asks open-ended questions, uses affirmations, engages in reflective listening and summarizes (Rollnick and Miller, 1995).

Some examples of how to do this are:

1   Open-ended questions which are questions that enable the person to talk about themselves and their perspective:
    • How has life been for you recently?
    • Could you describe how you are feeling?
    • What do you want to get out of me being here?
2   Reflective listening, which are statements by the nurse which show the client that you are attempting to understand their point of view:
    • So, I am hearing you feel frustrated that you will be on medication for the rest of your life.
    • I am not sure if I have this right. Are you angry that you take medication every day?
3   Affirmations are statements that reinforce messages of change from the client:
    • I can see at times that you have tried to work at taking your medication.
    • That sounds like the beginning of a good plan.
    • I can see how you have thought about the way you approach your medication and it looks like that would be a way to maintain taking your medication.
4   Summarizing captures brief periods of the interview and shows the client that the nurse has captured what has been said, felt and proposed during that time:
    • So, if I have this right, things haven't been going too well for you at the moment. You're feeling a bit frustrated that you may be on the medication for the rest of your life. At times you see that the medication is helpful and sometimes you're not too sure. From what you see, there are many people who have side effects of the medication and you are worried about this. At the moment you can't see any good reason for taking the medication.

The application of motivational interviewing technique was helpful for Paul, as initially he took his medication regularly and attended the men's group on a weekly basis, but then the situation started to change. Paul became quite ambivalent about taking his medication and would often miss doses. Staff at the men's group and Paul's

Table 3.1 Example of a training plan

Stage	One	Two	Three	Four	Five	Six
Topic	What is a psychosis	Medication	Recognizing signs and symptoms	Services	Support	Well-being and recovery
Learning points	Positive symptoms Negative symptoms Phases Common misunderstandings Individual stories	Types (anti-psychotic, benzodiazepines, etc.) Dosage Timing How medications work Side effects Long-term physical effects	Early warning signs Stress-vulnerability model Positive/negative signs Crisis phase	What's available Who to contact Self-help groups Psychological interventions Psychosocial interventions	How family can help Challenges that may arise How can learning be put into practice?	How to connect learning, being active and giving (nef, 2008) Creating a wrap Staying well

family had noticed that he was engaging less and tending to take himself away from social situations. By using a motivational interviewing approach it was established that Paul did not want to be on tablets all his life. On this basis the nurse explored how Paul felt when he was taking tablets and how he felt when he was not taking them, and a list of pros and cons of taking tablets was agreed. The nurse also directed Paul towards the evidence of the effectiveness of the medication he was receiving. Together they then formulated a care plan for the administration and monitoring of his medication.

NICE guidelines (2009) highlight the effectiveness of art therapy in the treatment of people with a psychosis. A study by Richardson et al. (2007) further indicates that art therapy could reduce negative symptoms. Using art therapy the mental health nurse works alongside the service user to identify activities, treatments, people, places, music and so on that contribute to keeping the service user well. A representative model or drawing is made of what has been identified, and placed in a box. While creating the object the nurse engages with the service user, using active listening skills to develop a sense of meaning for the person and to highlight when such things occur or if they are not present (Copeland, 1997).

Among many objects, Paul created a picture of a football to show how attending the match was a means of him keeping well. He copied the words to a song to show his taste in music and how he sometimes felt. The mental health nurse was able to engage with Paul using active listening skills. Paul was able to express what he got from attending the match (socialization, fun, camaraderie and emotional release). The mental health nurse was also able to talk with Paul about the meaning of the words to the song for Paul. Together they explored the notion of shyness and how Paul had felt different to others since his diagnosis of schizophrenia.

The protection shield can be used as a means of identifying the resources that the person has to enable recovery. As previously mentioned, within the recovery process, hope and resilience are two main factors in enabling recovery. Alongside the service user, the mental health nurse, using active listening skills, will facilitate the identification of factors that are protective for the person. Each factor should be given a representative drawing/object on paper or canvas. This enables the patient to identify within them what resources they have to prevent relapse.

Overall, Paul had many attributes which he identified as being able to protect him (Torgalsboen and Rund, 2010). He used a picture of the sea to represent his calmness and drew a picture of a book to resemble his education and knowledge. When talking with the mental health nurse, Paul was able to describe how being calm helped him take in information when having to make decisions. Paul also explained how his level of education had enabled him to build his knowledge of schizophrenia and take an active part in his treatment plan.

Summary of the key points

Mental health nurses utilizing psychological interventions should always seek to form a therapeutic alliance with the client, which is considerate of the service user's perspective and maintains the individual's narrative while treatment is being negotiated and then delivered.

Mental health service users should be recognized as having expertise in their condition.

Good and effective supervision needs to be sought when using cognitive behaviour therapy. The delivery of this approach should also be shaped by the process of recovery.

Psychological interventions delivered to mental health service users with a diagnosis of psychosis need to be holistic, which includes considering the physical health dimension. Maintaining well-being is equal to preventing ill mental health.

Quick quiz

1   Describe your understanding of the recovery process.
2   Identify the main theories relating to the causes of schizophrenia.
3   List the skills that a person who has a period of hospitalization may need on discharge.
4   Identify the key components of a learning set for families concerning psychosis.
5   Give an example of how you would negotiate a treatment plan with a person who has had an experience of psychosis.
6   Identify the four symptom categories of a psychosis.
7   Identify and explain a psychological intervention for people with a psychosis.
8   Give an example of how you would engage a person with schizophrenia using art therapy.
9   Motivational interviewing identifies a four-letter acronym for skills that nurses can employ. What is that acronym?
10   Give an example of one positive and one negative symptom of schizophrenia.

References

Addington, J. and Gleeson, J. (2005) Implementing cognitive–behavioural therapy for first-episode psychosis, *British Journal of Psychiatry*, 187(48): 72–6.

Akal, B.N. and Dogan, O. (2010) Potential risk factors for schizophrenia, *Archives of Neuropsychiatry*, 4: 230–6.

Ashir, M. and Marlowe, K. (2009) Traffic Lights: a practical risk management system for community early intervention in psychosis teams, *Clinical Governance: An International Journal*, 14(3): 226–35.

Bak, M., Myin-Qermeys, I., Hanssen, M., Bijl, R., Vollebergh, W., Delespaul, P. and Van Os, J. (2003) When does experience of psychosis result in a need for care? A prospective general population study, *Schizophrenia Bulletin*, 29(2): 349–58.

Barber, P. and Robertson, D. (2009) *Essential Pharmacology for Nurses*. Maidenhead: McGraw-Hill.

Barker, P.J. and Buchanan-Barker, P. (2005) *The Tidal Model: A Guide for Mental Health Professionals*. London: Brunner-Routledge.

Barrett, E.A., Sundet, K., Faerden, A., Nesvag, R., Agartz, I., Fosse, R., Mork, E., Steen, N., Andreassen, O.A. and Melle, I. (2010) Suicidality before and in the early phases of first episode psychosis, *Schizophrenia Research*, 119: 11–17.

Berry, K. and Haddock, G. (2008) The implementation of the NICE guidelines for schizophrenia: barriers to the implementation of psychological interventions and recommendations for the future, *Psychology and Psychotherapy: Theory, Research and Practice*, 81: 419–36.

Bird, V., Premkumar, P., Kendall, T., Whittington, C., Mitchell, J. and Kuipers, E. (2010) Early intervention services, cognitive-behavioural therapy and family intervention in early psychosis: systematic review, *British Journal of Psychiatry*, 197: 350–6.

Bracken, P. and Thomas, P. (2005) *Postpsychiatry: Mental Health in a Postmodern World.* Oxford: Oxford University Press.

Burton, N.L. (2006) *Psychiatry.* Oxford: Blackwell.

Comer, R.J. (2008) *Fundamentals of Abnormal Psychology*, 5th edn. New York: Worth.

Copeland, M.E. (1997) *Wellness Recovery Action Plan.* Dummerston: Peach Press.

Davey, G. (2008) *Psychopathology: Research, Assessment and Treatment in Clinical Psychology.* Oxford: Wiley-Blackwell.

Deegan, P. (1996) Recovery as a journey of the heart, *Psychiatric Rehabilitation Journal*, 19(3): 91–7.

Department of Health (DoH) (2006a) *From Values to Action: The Chief Nursing Officer's Review of Mental Health Nursing.* London: Department of Health.

Department of Health (DoH) (2006b) *Best Practice Competencies and Capabilities for Pre-registration Mental Health Nurses in England: The Chief Nursing Officer's Review of Mental Health Nursing.* London: Department of Health.

Department of Health (DoH) (2009) *New Horizons: A Shared Vision for Mental Health.* London: Department of Health.

Dixon, L.B. and Lehman, A.F. (1995) Family interventions for schizophrenia, *Schizophrenia Bulletin*, 21(4): 631–43.

Eales, S. (2009) Risk assessment and management, in P. Callaghan, J. Playle and L. Cooper (eds) *Mental Health Nursing Skills.* Oxford: Oxford University Press.

Frere, F. (2010) On the impact of being diagnosed with schizophrenia, *Journal of Mental Health*, 19(4): 376–8.

Fung, K.M.T., Tsang, H.W.H. and Corrigan, P.W. (2008) Self-stigma of people with schizophrenia as predictor of their adherence to psychosocial treatment, *Psychiatric Rehabilitation Journal*, 32(2): 95–104.

Gillam, T. and Williams, R. (2008) Understanding schizophrenia: a guide for newly qualified community nurses, *British Journal of Community Nursing*, 13(2): 84–8.

Hamilton, B. and Roper, C. (2006) Troubling 'insight': power and possibilities in mental health care, *Journal of Psychiatric and Mental Health Nursing*, 13: 416–22.

International Early Psychosis Writing Group (2005) International clinical practice guidelines for early psychosis, *British Journal of Psychiatry*, 187(48): 120–4.

Kuller, A.M., Tot, B.D., Goisman, R.M., Wainwright, L.D. and Rabin, R.J. (2010) Cognitive behavioral therapy and schizophrenia: a survey of clinical practices and views on efficacy in the United States and United Kingdom, *Community Mental Health Journal*, 46: 2–9.

Lester, H.E., Tritter, J.Q. and Sorohan, H. (2005) Patients' and health professionals' views on primary care for people with serious mental illness: focus group study, *BMJ: British Medical Journal*, 330(7500): 1122–6.

Lovejoy, M. (1984) Recovery from schizophrenia: a personal odyssey, *Hospital and Community Psychiatry*, 35: 809–12.

Mackeith, J. and Burns, S. (2008) *Mental Health Recovery Star: User Guide*. London: Mental Health Providers Forum and Triangle Consulting.

Merleau-Ponty, M. ([1945]1962) the body as expression and speech, in *The Phenomenology of Perception*, C. Smith, trans. 1962. London: Routledge.

Miller, W.R. (1983) Motivational interviewing with problem drinkers, *Behavioural Psychotherapy*, 11: 147–72.

Miller, W.R. and Rollnick, S. (1991) *Motivational Interviewing: Preparing People to Change Addictive Behaviour*. London: Guildford Press.

National Institute for Clinical Excellence (NICE) (2002) *Schizophrenia: Core Interventions in the Treatment and Management of Schizophrenia in Primary and Secondary Care*. London: National Institute for Clinical Excellence.

National Institute for Health and Clinical Excellence (NICE) (2009) *Schizophrenia: Core Interventions in the Treatment and Management of Schizophrenia in Adults in Primary and Secondary Care* (update of NICE clinical guideline 1). London: National Institute for Health and Clinical Excellence.

New Economics Foundation (nef) (2008) *Five Ways to Well-being: The Evidence*. London: New Economics Foundation.

Pandya, S. (2009) Antipsychotics: uses, actions and p   ribing rationale, *Nurse Prescribing*, 7(1): 23–7.

Pilling, S. and Price, K. (2006) Developing and implementing clinical guidelines: lessons from the NICE schizophrenia guideline, *Epidemiologia e Psichiatria Sociale*, 15(2): 109–16.

Pradesky, C. and Greenberger, D. (1995) *A Clinician's Guide to Mind over Mood*. New York: Guilford.

Prytys, M., Garety, P.A., Jolley, S., Onwumere, J. and Craig, T. (2011) Implementing the NICE guideline for schizophrenia recommendations for psychological therapies: a qualitative analysis of the attitudes of CMHT staff, *Clinical Psychology and Psychotherapy*, 18: 48–59.

Rapp, C.A. and Goscha, R. (2006) *The Strengths Model: Case Management and People with Psychiatric Disabilities*, 2nd edn. New York: Oxford University Press.

Richardson, P., Jones, K., Evans, C., Stevens, P. and Rowe, A. (2007) Exploratory RCT of art therapy as an adjunctive treatment in schizophrenia, *Journal of Mental Health*, 16(4): 483–91.

Rollnick, S. and Miller, W.R. (1995) What is motivational interviewing? *Behaviour and Cognitive Psychotherapy*, 23: 325–34.

Rusch, N. and Corrigan, P.W. (2002) Motivational interviewing to improve insight and treatment adherence in schizophrenia, *Psychiatric Rehabilitation Journal*, 26(1): 23–32.

Sadock, B.J. and Sadock, V.A. (2010) *Kaplan and Sadock's Pocket Handbook of Clinical Psychiatry*, 5th edn. London: Lippincott Williams & Wilkins.

Shepherd, S., Boardman, J. and Slade, M. (2008) *Making Recovery a Reality*. London: Sainsbury Centre for Mental Health.

Torgalsboen, A.K. and Rund, R.R. (2010) Maintenance of recovery from schizophrenia at 20 year follow up: what happened, *Psychiatry*, 73(1): 70–83.

Van Os, J. and Kapur, S. (2009) Schizophrenia, *Lancet*, 374: 635–4.

Westbrook, D., Kennerley, H. and Kirk, J. (2007) *An Introduction to Cognitive Behavioural Therapy*. London: Sage Publications.

4 Psychological interventions in anxiety and depression

Lisa Woods

Chapter aim and objectives

Aim
- To explore the nurse's role in relation to psychological interventions for anxiety and depression.

Objectives
- To provide an overview of anxiety and depression.
- To consider the management of psychological interventions for individuals with anxiety and depression.
- To highlight the relevant evidenced-based practice guidance for working with individuals with anxiety and depression.
- To identify key psychological interventions for individuals with anxiety and depression.

What are anxiety and depression?

Depression is a mood disorder; it refers to a range of mental health problems determined by the lowering of mood and loss of interest or pleasure in usual activities. People experience a range of associated cognitive, behavioural and autonomic symptoms which can typically include lack of interest or pleasure, reduced energy, decrease in activity, reduced concentration and attention, marked tiredness after even minimum effort, poor appetite and disturbed sleep. People often experience feelings of guilt or worthlessness, reduced self-esteem and self-confidence and thoughts of death or suicide (WHO, 1992; APA, 2000).

A diagnosis of depression relates to the number and severity of symptoms that a person presents with. Depression may be defined as mild (minor functional impairment), moderate (functional impairment that is between mild and severe and difficulty in maintaining daily activities) or severe (persistent low mood with symptoms that are marked and distressing). Depression can be classified as a single depressive episode or a recurrent depressive disorder. Depression is seen as recurrent if the person has experienced two or more depressive episodes. Severe depression can also occur with psychotic symptoms, this is when the person also experiences hallucinations, delusion, psychomotor retardation or stupor (WHO, 1992; APA, 2000).

Anxiety is a disorder in which a person predominately experiences a persistent feeling of dread, apprehension, tension, uneasiness or impending disaster (Churchill et al., 2009). The definition anxiety disorder covers a number of disorders where the primary feature is abnormal or inappropriate anxiety. The major types of anxiety disorder are generalized anxiety disorder (GAD) (generalized and persistent 'free-floating' anxiety most of the time), panic disorder (recurrent severe anxiety/panic attacks that are often unpredictable; this can be with or without agoraphobia), phobia (fear and panic in specific situations or with objects such as animals, heights and enclosed spaces), social phobia (fear of scrutiny by other people, leading to avoidance of social situations), obsessive compulsive disorder (recurrent obsessional thoughts or compulsive acts in order to prevent harm to the individual or someone else), post-traumatic stress disorder (a delayed or protracted response to a stressful event or situation of an exceptionally threatening or catastrophic nature) and acute stress reaction (a brief stress reaction after exposure to an extreme traumatic stress) (WHO, 1992; APA, 2000).

Anxiety is associated with a number of cognitive, behavioural and autonomic symptoms including worry, irritability, poor concentration, increased sensitivity to noise, sleep disturbance, sweating, dry mouth, palpitations, urinary frequency, gastric problems, hyperventilation, shortness of breath and dizziness, increased muscle tension, restlessness, inability to relax, headaches and aching pains, particularly in the shoulders and back.

It is not uncommon for people to experience symptoms of depression and anxiety at the same time. If this occurs a diagnosis of mixed depression and anxiety can be made. Kroenke et al. (2007) found that people who experience mixed depression and anxiety have a worse prognosis, increased associated disability and more persistent symptoms than when someone experiences either depression or anxiety alone.

There are two classification systems for mental disorders: *The ICD–10 Classification of Mental and Behavioural Disorders* (ICD–10) (WHO, 1992) and *Diagnostic and Statistical Manual of Mental Disorders* of the American Psychiatric Association (DSM–IV-TR) (APA, 2000). Both systems are similar and overlap in terms of disorders and symptoms of anxiety and depression, however definitions of severity differ. For example, DSM–IV-TR (APA, 2000) now recognizes sub-threshold depression and generalized anxiety disorder, in which a person may not meet the full criteria for the disorder but can experience some depressive or anxiety symptoms that can affect their quality of life and level of functioning (NICE, 2009; 2011).

The prevalence of depression and anxiety disorders in the general population is significant; 6 million people in the UK experience common mental health problems, of which over half of these suffer from depression or anxiety. At least one in four people will experience a mental health problem at some point in their life and, at any given time, one in six adults is experiencing depression or anxiety, with almost half of all adults experiencing at least one episode of depression during their lifetime. Ten per cent of children have a diagnosable mental health condition and 50 per cent of lifetime mental illness is present by the age of 14 (Andrews et al., 2005; McManus et al., 2009). Globally in 2000 depression was the leading cause of disability measured by years lost due to disability and the fourth leading contributor to the burden of disease.

However, statistics have projected that by 2020 depression will have accelerated to be the second leading contributor to the global burden of disease internationally for all ages and for both sexes (WHO, 2011).

The personal costs of mental health problems are far reaching; they cause distress not only to the individual but also to their families and friends, and can impact upon local communities. Mental health problems affect a person's social and occupational functioning, physical health, mortality and morbidity (DH, 2011a). Moussavi et al. (2007) report that depression and anxiety cause a greater deterioration in state of health than the major chronic physical illnesses, that is, angina, arthritis, asthma and diabetes. Therefore, providing interventions that can improve mental health can positively influence outcomes across a wide range of domains, including lifestyles, physical health, recovery, employment and earnings, and improved quality of life (Friedli, 2009).

A World Health Organization international study (Moussavi et al., 2007) found that depression alone produced a significantly greater deterioration in a person's overall health and functioning compared with the effects of a range of chronic conditions, such as angina, asthma, diabetes and arthritis. The study also reported that co-morbidity with depression and a chronic disease significantly worsened a person's state of health. The co-morbidity of depression and anxiety in physical illness is well recognized and studies have consistently shown the relationships between depressive and anxiety disorders and a wide range of chronic physical conditions (Scott et al., 2007; DH, 2011).

Stigma surrounding mental health conditions can be due to the widespread misconceptions about their causes and nature. Mental health conditions often are seen by individuals and society as personal weakness (WHO, 2010). For people experiencing mental health problems there continue to be social exclusion and health inequalities in areas of their life such as housing, education and employment, as well as in social and family relationships.

Suicide accounts for nearly 1 per cent of all deaths in the general population, however nearly two-thirds of this figure occurs in people with depression; significant risk factors for eventual suicide being the severity of depression, hopelessness and suicidal idealization (Brown et al., 2000). Please see Chapter 1 for further information in relation to risk and the new cross-government suicide prevention strategy which is due to be published in 2011. The following two scenarios provide an overview of the impact of common mental health problems, the issues arising will be dealt with in more depth in the psychological interventions section.

SCENARIO 1

Joe is a 49-year-old man referred to the crisis team following an assessment by his GP. Joe was made redundant six months previously and has been unable to find another job. He told his GP that he can't cope any more; he hates himself and the person he has become over the past few months.

(continued)

Joe has had a history of depressive episodes for most of his adult life. He described his first period of depression as a 'total breakdown' after failing his exams at college. Joe has been prescribed several different antidepressants over the years and has had one short in-patient admission 10 years ago following a suicide attempt.

During the crisis team assessment Joe described several symptoms of low mood, difficulty falling asleep and waking around 5 a.m. worrying about money and his family. He described feeling tired all the time and having little energy or motivation, even to get washed and dressed in the mornings. He said he is doing very little at the moment and is struggling to concentrate on the television or conversations with his family; he has been avoiding people, even avoiding spending time with his grandchildren, which he feels very guilty about. Joe said that he can't see the point in thinking about his future any more, everything seems hopeless. He has had thoughts that he wishes he wasn't here any more; he had not made any plans or taken any actions to kill himself but prayed that he wouldn't wake up in the morning. He believed that he had let his family down and they would be better off without him.

SCENARIO 2

Jessica is a 22-year-old woman who described experiencing symptoms of anxiety on and off since the age of 14 years. Jessica was originally seen by a counsellor at her GP surgery at the age of 16, she was then referred to the adult mental health service by her GP but frequently missed appointments and was discharged. Jessica has recently been re-referred and has now had two routine outpatient appointments with a consultant psychiatrist.

Since the age of 14 years Jessica has been offered a range of support to help manage her symptoms of anxiety; this has included medication, relaxation training and individual appointments with a GP-based counsellor. Jessica described her symptoms as anxiety and worry about a variety of situations. She has significant difficulty in controlling the anxiety and worry, and finds it very difficult to regain control and relax when she starts to worry. She described feeling restless, tension in her muscles, concentration problems, irritability and difficulty sleeping. Jessica was very distressed as her anxiety was affecting every aspect of her daily life and she just wanted to be happy.

Evidence-based practice

Mental health nurses at the point of registration must have the knowledge, skills and behaviours to improve the health and well-being of service users. They must have the ability to access and utilize the best available evidence and technology to deliver complex care to a high standard and enhance the quality of mental health service provision (NMC, 2010).

There is now a significant body of evidence-based psychological interventions demonstrating efficacy in the treatment of depression and anxiety disorders. The evidence, however, reflects the broad range of psychological therapies and demonstrates varying levels of efficacy dependent on the therapy and the severity of symptoms. Some psychological therapies, although well established, lack the research evidence to support their efficacy. Lack of research does not necessarily mean the therapy is ineffective, but does mean that national guidance such as that issued by the National Institute of Clinical Excellence (NICE) and Cochrane reviews cannot make evidence-based recommendations and guide service provision regarding treatments and care when research is limited.

Roth and Fonagy (2005) differentiate psychological therapies under the following broad headings:

- behavioural or cognitive behavioural therapies
- counselling
- interpersonal therapy (IPT)
- group therapy
- psychodynamic therapy
- supportive and experiential therapy
- systemic therapy.

The mental health strategy *No Health Without Mental Health* (DH, 2011a; 2011b) states that a key area for action is to ensure that all people with mental health problems are offered age and developmentally appropriate information,   nd a choice of high-quality evidence and practice-based interventions, including   chological therapies. Specifically, the government is committed to ensuring that all adults with depression and anxiety will have access to a choice of psychological therapies and an expansion of psychological therapies for children and young people, older adults and their carers, people with severe mental illness, physical long-term conditions and medically unexplained symptoms (DH, 2011b).

Only one in four adults experiencing depression or anxiety are receiving any kind of treatment (Centre for Economic Performance's Mental Health Policy Group, 2006; McManus et al., 2009). Although most service users preferred psychological interventions to medication (Prins et al., 2008), the most common form of treatment is medication only, followed eventually by psychological intervention alone or in combination with medication. Psychological therapies are not readily available for all due to the limited number of trained physiological therapists. Waiting lists for therapy can be over nine months, if a therapist is available at all, and therefore often the treatment offered is medication alone.

NICE (2009) also reported that people are not seeking timely help for depressive and anxiety symptoms owing to their reluctance to ask for help and the failure of health professionals to recognize mental health problems, particularly in primary care. Meltzer et al. (2000) found the two most frequent reasons for people resisting seeking help were the belief that no one could help and that people felt they should be able to cope with their problems themselves.

In response to the national demand to expand the provision of mental health care and psychological therapies for people with mental health problems, a national programme, Improving Access to Psychological Therapies (IAPT), was established in 2008. A key aim of the programme was to develop a competent workforce to deliver evidence-based, NICE-approved psychological therapies and interventions (primarily for people with anxiety and depression) to promote recovery and help people return to full social and occupational functioning (DH, 2008a; 2008b).

A 'stepped care' model (Figure 4.1) of health-care delivery has been designed which considers the severity of a person's depression and anxiety alongside the evidence base and choice of intervention and service depending on that severity. The model considers the relationship between primary and secondary care service in its management of people with mental health problems. The model recommends the least intensive or intrusive interventions should be offered first, which are likely to produce a significant health gain (Bower and Gilbody, 2005; NICE, 2009; 2011). In order for a 'stepped care' model to be effective, Bower and Gilbody (2005) state it is crucial that the model is 'self-correcting', in that the progress and outcome of each intervention are monitored and systematically evaluated. Should the first intervention/step not prove to produce a significant health gain, then it is the responsibility of the health practitioner to initiate collaborative changes and consider 'stepping up' the plan of care at the earliest opportunity.

NICE guidelines have reviewed the evidence for the effectiveness of a range of psychological interventions in the treatment of mild, moderate and severe depression and anxiety disorders. Cognitive behavioural therapy (CBT) or interventions based on the theoretical underpinnings of CBT are recommended as superior in terms of treatment choice (NICE, 2005a; 2005b; 2009; 2011). The majority of evidence has been undertaken however with working-age adults; therefore care must be taken in generalizing what evidence there is to other clinical populations such as older adults and children (Wilson et al., 2008). NICE recommends low-intensity interventions based on the principles of CBT for mild to moderate depression and most anxiety disorders. Recommended intervention-specific and problem-specific interventions include guided self-help, non-facilitated self-help, behavioural activation, cognitive restructuring, problem-solving and exposure (NICE, 2005a; 2005b; 2009; 2011; Hunot et al., 2007; Roth and Pilling, 2007; Richards, 2010).

For moderate and severe anxiety or depressive disorders and people who have not responded to initial low-intensity psychological interventions (see stepped care model, Figure 4.1) several psychological therapies are recommended due to their level of efficacy. CBT and IPT have the strongest evidence base, and behavioural activation is also suggested; however, the evidence is less robust. In addition, behavioural couples therapy is advocated if beneficial to the person's relationship and contributing to their depression. For anxiety disorders CBT is seen as superior to other therapies, however both applied relaxation, psychodynamic therapies are recommended in the treatment of GAD, and eye movement desensitization and reprocessing (EMDR) in the treatment of PTSD (NICE, 2005a; 2005b; 2009; 2011; Hunot et al., 2007; Roth and Pilling, 2007).

Based on the limited evidence base of psychological intervention for children and young people, for mild depression NICE (2005c) recommends non-directive supportive therapy, group CBT or guided self-help. For severe depression it recommends individual CBT, interpersonal therapy or shorter-term family therapy (see also Chapter 10).

Focus of the intervention	Nature of the intervention
STEP 4: Severe and complex depression, treatment refractory GAD; marked functional impairment; risk to life; severe self-neglect	Highly specialist treatment, complex drug and/or psychological treatment, crisis service, combined treatments, multiprofessional and in-patient care
STEP 3: Persistent sub-threshold depressive symptoms or mild to moderate depression or GAD with inadequate response to initial interventions; moderate and severe depression GAD	Medication, high-intensity psychological interventions, combined treatments, collaborative care and referral for further assessment and interventions
STEP 2: Persistent sub-threshold depressive symptoms; mild to moderate depression or GAD that has not improved after education and active monitoring in primary care	Low-intensity psychological and psychosocial interventions, medication individual guided self-help and psychoeducation, and referral for further assessment and interventions
STEP 1: All known and suspected presentations of depression and anxiety	Assessment, support, psychoeducation, active monitoring and referral for further assessment and interventions

Figure 4.1 A model of 'stepped care'

A psychological intervention often offered for depression and anxiety disorders is counselling, particularly within a primary care setting. The robust evidence base for counselling is limited and therefore it is not mentioned extensively in the NICE guidelines for depression and GAD/panic disorder. There is research to support the efficacy of counselling, such as a Cochrane review which found counselling more effective than usual care in reducing psychological symptoms in the short term but it appeared to provide no additional advantage in long-term care (Bower and Rowland, 2006).

In addition to psychological interventions, pharmacological treatments are also recommended in depression and anxiety disorders. For mild to moderate depression or anxiety, where no treatment has previously been offered, the choice of either psychological or pharmacological treatment should be based on a person's preference as there is no significant evidence that either mode of treatment is better. However, for moderate or severe depression and anxiety a combination of medication and psychological intervention is often recommended for treatment efficacy (Perlis et al., 2002; NICE, 2005a; 2005b; 2009; 2011; Bortolotti et al., 2008).

Psychological interventions and scenarios

The standards for pre-registration nursing (NMC, 2010) state that mental health nurses must be competent in applying their knowledge and skills in a range of psychological interventions. While pre-registration mental health nursing does not aspire to produce psychological therapists, a core requirement for all mental health nurses is to promote mental health and well-being, through acquiring knowledge of and competence in evidence-based psychological interventions which can enable people to recover from their mental distress (DH, 2006a; 2006b).

Nurses will work with individuals with mild, moderate and severe depression and anxiety disorders at any step of the stepped care model. While only post-qualifying training programmes can enable nurses to become psychological therapists, pre-registration nursing programmes should include training in certain psychological and psychosocial interventions for anxiety and depression. Roth and Pilling (2007) specify that it is vital to guide and structure the type and level of psychological and psychosocial interventions taught to pre-registration nurses. Training should be based on evidence-based frameworks and competences in order to ensure well-delivered, problem-specific, psychological interventions. Alongside problem-specific intervention training, several generic competencies should also be taught, such as engagement skills as the technical skills of specific interventions are unlikely to be successful if the nurse does not spend time building a trusting therapeutic relationship with the service user (see also Chapter 2).

It is critical that nurses undertaking psychological interventions have in-depth knowledge of mental health problems, an understanding of and ability to operate within professional and ethical guidelines, and can understand and apply knowledge underpinning the model of the psychological interventions they are undertaking (Roth and Pilling, 2007) (see also Chapter 11). Based on information discussed in the evidence-based section, nursing guidance and competency frameworks for anxiety and depression as a range of psychological and psychosocial interventions could be taught as part of pre-registration mental health nursing curriculum. Evidence-based psychological interventions specifically focusing on treatments to address clearly defined problems and behaviours and enhance psychological skills and well-being are:

- cognitive restructuring
- behavioural activation
- problem solving

- relapse prevention
- psychosocial interventions
- motivational interviewing
- guided self-help
- exposure (NICE, 2005a; 2005b; 2009; 2011; DH, 2006a; Roth and Pilling, 2007; Bennett-Levy et al., 2010; NMC, 2010; Richards, 2010).

Alongside formal diagnostic criteria DSM–IV or ICD–10 used by medical staff, a range of psychometric measures can be used by nurses to help identify if someone is experiencing anxiety or depression and the severity of symptoms experienced. A number of measures have been produced, the most frequently used validated tools are the Patient Health Questionnaire (PHQ-9) (Spitzer et al., 1999), the Beck Depression Inventory (BDI) (Beck et al., 1996), Generalized Anxiety Disorder assessment (GAD-7) (Spitzer et al., 2006), Hospital Anxiety and Depression Scale (HADS) (Zigmond and Snaith, 1983), Beck Anxiety Inventory (BAI) (Beck et al., 1988) and the General Health Questionnaire (GHQ) (Goldberg and Williams, 1991).

SCENARIO 1

Joe was referred for psychological therapy by the crisis team. Following assessment and while waiting for cognitive behavioural therapy, the psychological therapy service recommended that a nurse within the crisis team commence behavioural activation with Joe to help establish activities that Joe has stopped doing and to slowly reintroduce routine, pleasurable and necessary activities back into his day.

Behavioural activation is a discrete, time-limited, structured psychological intervention. It is an effective treatment as it targets the role of avoidance in depression. Behavioural activation focuses on activities to help service users re-establish daily routines, increase pleasurable activities and address important necessary issues that people commonly avoid when feeling depressed (Richards and Whyte, 2009; NICE, 2010). Evidence has shown that behavioural activation has been found to increase subjective well-being, including levels of happiness and satisfaction in life of individuals with clinical and symptoms of depression (Mazzucchelli et al., 2010).

The nurse followed an evidence-based treatment framework to help direct the structure and duration of the intervention with Joe:

Step 1: Explaining behavioural activation
Step 2: Identifying routine, pleasurable and necessary activities
Step 3: Making a hierarchy of routine, pleasurable and necessary activities
Step 4: Planning some routine, pleasurable and necessary activities
Step 5: Implementing behavioural activation exercises
Step 6: Reviewing progress
(Lovell and Richards, 2008; Richards and Whyte, 2009)

SCENARIO 2

Following a comprehensive reassessment of Jessica's anxiety symptoms and previous treatments, the psychiatrist decided that although Jessica had been offered treatments by mental health services on a number of occasions, she had not received the most appropriate treatment to effectively manage her symptoms of anxiety. Based on the stepped care model of interventions for anxiety, the psychiatrist discharged Jessica back to primary care mental health services to receive the most appropriate intervention that was likely to improve her symptoms of generalised anxiety disorder.

Owing to Jessica's level of symptoms and function impairment it was decided that she would benefit from cognitive behavioural interventions (step 3) (NICE, 2011). Step three psychological interventions should be facilitated by an appropriately trained psychological therapist, however alongside such interventions and in collaboration with the psychological therapist, problem-specific interventions may be beneficial to help reduce symptoms that a service user may be experiencing. Jessica identified a significant problem with her sleep which was compounding her anxiety symptoms. The nurse within the primary care service followed a treatment framework to help direct the structure and duration of the sleep management intervention with Jessica:

Step 1: Establish the nature of the service user's sleep difficulties
Step 2: Provide information about normal sleep and the nature of sleep problems
Step 3: Provide information on sleep hygiene and encourage the service user to establish regular sleep routines
Step 4: Monitor the effects of the above

Summary of the key points

The prevalence of depression and anxiety disorders in the general population is significant; severity of symptoms can vary from mild to severe, single episode to recurrent illness. There is an increasing body of evidence-based psychological interventions demonstrating efficacy in the treatment of depression and anxiety disorders. The evidence, however, reflects the broad range of psychological therapies, and demonstrates varying levels of efficacy dependent on the therapy and the severity of symptoms.

The standards for pre-registration nursing education (NMC, 2010) state that nurses should be competent in a range of evidence-based psychological and psychosocial individual and group interventions at the point of registration. They must have the ability to access and utilize the best available evidence and technology to deliver complex care to a high standard and enhance the quality of mental health service provision.

While pre-registration nursing training does not intend to produce psychological thera-pists, nurses need to develop skills to deliver certain psychological and psychosocial interventions. To ensure competence in the interventions, nurses should under-take appropriate training in their delivery, receive regular high-quality supervision, use routine outcome measures to monitor and evaluate the efficacy of the treat-ment and have managerial support to undertake this role (DH, 2006b; NICE, 2009; 2011; National IAPT Programme, 2011).

Quick quiz

1   Define depression.
2   Define anxiety.
3   What is the stepped care model?
4   What step of the model should Joe be on?
5   What step of the model should Jessica be on?
6   What interventions does NICE recommend for mild, moderate and severe anxiety?
7   What interventions does NICE recommend for mild, moderate and severe depression?
8   What do the standards for pre-registration nursing education say in relation to competency and psychological and psychosocial interventions?

References

American Psychiatric Association (APA) (2000) *Diagnostic and Statistical Manual of Mental Disorders*, 4th edn text revision (DSM–IV-TR). Washington, DC: APA.

Andrews, G., Poulton, R. and Skoog, I. (2005) Lifetime risk of depression: restricted to a minority or waiting for most? *British Journal of Psychiatry*, 187: 495–6.

Beck, A.T., Epstein, N., Brown, G. and Steer, R.A. (1988) An inventory of measuring anxiety: psychometric properties, *Journal of Consulting and Clinical Psychology*, 56: 893–7.

Beck, A.T., Steer, A. and Brown, G.K. (1996) *Beck Depression Inventory Manual*, 2nd edn. San Antonio, TX: Psychological Corporation.

Bennett-Levy, J., Richards, D. and Farrand, P. (2010) Low intensity CBT interventions: a revolution in mental health, in J. Bennett-Levy, D. Richards, P. Farrand, H. Christensen, K. Griffiths, D.J. Kavanagh, B. Klein, M.A. Lau, J. Proudfoot, L. Ritterband, J. White and C. Williams (eds) (2010) *Oxford Guide to Low Intensity CBT Interventions*. Oxford: Oxford University Press.

Bortolotti, B., Menchetti, M., Bellini, F., Montaguti, M.B. and Berardi, D. (2008) Psycho-logical interventions for major depression in primary care: a meta-analytic review of randomized controlled trials, *General Hospital Psychiatry*, 30(4): 293–302.

Bower, P. and Gilbody, S. (2005) Stepped care in psychological therapies: access, effectiveness and efficiency, *British Journal of Psychiatry*, 186: 11–17.

Bower, P.J. and Rowland, N. (2006) Effectiveness and cost effectiveness of counselling in primary care, *Cochrane Database of Systematic Reviews*, issue 3.

Brown, G.K., Beck, A.T., Steer, R.A. and Grisham, J.R. (2000) Risk factors for suicide in psychiatric outpatients: a 20 year prospective study, *Journal of Consulting and Clinical Psychology*, 68(3): 371–7.

Centre for Economic Performance's Mental Health Policy Group (2006) *The Depression Report: A New Deal for Depression and Anxiety Disorders*. London: LSE.

Churchill, R., Barbui, C., Caldwell, D., Cipriani, A., Furukawa, T., Gilbody, S., Hazel, P., Hetrick, S., Hunot, V., Ipser, J., Jackson, D., Lam, R., Lewis, G., Simon, G. and Turner, R. (2009) *Cochrane Depression, Anxiety and Neurosis Group: About the Cochrane Collaboration (Cochrane Review Groups (CRGs))*, issue 2.

Department of Health (DH) (2006a) *Best Practice Competencies and Capabilities for Pre-registration Mental Health Nurses in England: The Chief Nursing Officer's Review of Mental Health Nursing*. London: Department of Health.

Department of Health (DH) (2006b) *From Values to Action: The Chief Nursing Officer's Review of Mental Health Nursing*. London: Department of Health.

Department of Health (DH) (2008a) *IAPT Implementation Plan: National Guidelines for Regional Delivery*. London: Department of Health.

Department of Health (DH) (2008b) *Commissioning IAPT for the Whole Community: Improving Access to Psychological Therapies*. London: Department of Health.

Department of Health (DH) (2011a) *No Health Without Mental Health: A Cross-government Mental Health Outcomes Strategy for People of All Ages*. London: HMG/DH.

Department of Health (DH) (2011b) *Talking Therapies: A Four-year Plan of Action: A Supporting Document to No Health Without Mental Health: A Cross-government Mental Health Outcomes Strategy for People of All Ages*. London: Department of Health.

Friedli, L. (2009) *Mental Health, Resilience and Inequalities*. Copenhagen: World Health Organization.

Goldberg, D.P. and Williams, P. (1991) *A User's Guide to the General Health Questionnaire*. Windsor: NFER-Nelson.

Hunot, V., Churchill, R., Teixeira, V. and Silva de Lima, M. (2007) Psychological therapies for generalised anxiety disorder, *Cochrane Database of Systematic Reviews*, issue 1.

Kroenke, K., Spitzer, R.L., Williams, J.B., Monahan, P. O. and Lowe, B. (2007) Anxiety disorders in primary care: prevalence, impairment, co-morbidity, and detection, *Annals of Internal Medicine*, 146: 317–25.

Lovell, K. and Richards, D. (2008) *A Recovery Programme for Depression*. London: Rethink.

Mazzucchelli, T.G., Kane, R.T. and Rees, C.S. (2010) Behavioural activation interventions for well-being: a meta-analysis, *Journal of Positive Psychology*, 5(2): 105–21.

McManus, S., Meltzer, H. and Brugha, T. (2009) *Adult Psychiatric Morbidity in England, 2007: Results of a Household Survey*. Leeds: NHS Information Centre for Health and Social Care.

Meltzer, H., Bebbington, P. and Brugha, T. (2000) The reluctance to seek treatment for neurotic disorders, *Journal of Mental Health*, 9: 319–27.

Mousavi, S., Chatterji, S., Verdes, E., Tandon, A., Patel, V. and Ustun, B. (2007) Depression, chronic diseases, and decrements in health: results from the World Health Surveys, *Lancet*, 370: 851–8.

National IAPT Programme (2011) *Which Talking Therapy for Depression? A Guide to Understanding the Different Psychological Therapies you may be Offered to Treat your Depression*. London: Department of Health.

National Institute of Clinical Excellence (NICE) (2005a) *Post-traumatic Stress Disorder (PTSD): The Management of PTSD in Adults and Children in Primary and Secondary Care.* London: British Psychological Society and Royal College of Psychiatrists.

National Institute of Clinical Excellence (NICE) (2005b) *Obsessive-compulsive Disorder: Core Interventions in the Treatment of Obsessive-compulsive Disorder and Body Dysmorphic Disorder.* London: British Psychological Society and Royal College of Psychiatrists.

National Institute of Clinical Excellence (NICE) (2005c) *Depression in Children and Young People: Full Guidance.* London: British Psychological Society and Royal College of Psychiatrists.

National Institute of Clinical Excellence (NICE) (2009) *The Treatment and Management of Depression in Adults,* updated edn. London: British Psychological Society and Royal College of Psychiatrists.

National Institute of Clinical Excellence (NICE) (2011) *Generalised Anxiety Disorder and Panic Disorder (With or Without Agoraphobia) in Adults: Management in Primary, Secondary and Community Care,* partial update. London: British Psychological Society and Royal College of Psychiatrists.

Nursing Midwifery Council (NMC) (2010) *Standards for Pre-registration Nursing Education.* London: Nursing Midwifery Council.

Perlis, R.H., Nierenberg, A.A., Alpert, J.E., Pava, J., Matthews, J.D., Buchin, J., Sickinger, A.H. and Fava, M. (2002) Effects of adding cognitive therapy to fluoxetine dose increase on risk of relapse and residual depressive symptoms in continuation treatment of major depressive disorder, *Journal of Clinical Psychopharmacology,* 22: 474–80.

Prins, M.A., Verhaak, P.F.M., Bensing, J.M. and Van der Meer, K. (2008) Health beliefs and perceived need for mental health care of anxiety and depression: the patient's perspective explored, *Clinical Psychology Review,* 28: 1038–58.

Richards, D. (2010) Behavioural activation for depression, in J. Bennett-Levy, D. Richards, P. Farrand, H. Christensen, K. Griffiths, D.J. Kavanagh, B. Klein, M.A. Lau, J. Proudfoot, L. Ritterband, J. White and C. Williams (eds) (2010) *Oxford Guide to Low Intensity CBT Interventions.* Oxford: Oxford University Press.

Richards, D. and Whyte, M. (2009) *Reach Out: National Programme Educators Materials to Support the Delivery of Training for Psychological Wellbeing Practitioners Delivering Low Intensity Interventions,* 2nd edn. London: Rethink.

Roth, A. and Fonagy, P. (2005) *What Works for Whom: A Critical Review of Psychotherapy Research,* 2nd edn. New York: Guilford.

Roth, A.D. and Pilling, S. (2007) *The Competences Required to Deliver Effective Cognitive and Behavioural Therapy for People with Depression and with Anxiety Disorders.* London: Department of Health.

Scott, K.M., Bruffaerts, R., Tsang, A., Ormel, J., Alonso, J., Angermeye, M.C., Benjet, C. et al. (2007) Depression–anxiety relationships with chronic physical conditions: results from the World Mental Health Surveys, *Journal of Affective Disorders,* 103(1–3): 113–20.

Spitzer, R.L., Kroenke, K., Williams, J.B. and Lowe, B. (2006) A brief measure for assessing generalized anxiety disorder: the GAD-7, *Archives of Internal Medicine,* 22(10): 1092–7.

Spitzer, R.L., Kroenke, K., Williams, J.B. and Patient Health Questionnaire Primary Care Study Group (1999) Validation and utility of a self-report version of PRIME-MD: the PHQ primary care study, *Journal of the American Medical Association,* 282: 1737–44.

Wilson, K., Mottram, P.G. and Vassilas, C. (2008) Psychotherapeutic treatments for older depressed people, *Cochrane Database of Systematic Reviews*, issue 1.

World Health Organization (WHO) (1992) *The ICD–10 Classification of Mental and Behavioural Disorders: Clinical Descriptions and Diagnostic Guidelines*. Geneva: WHO.

World Health Organization (WHO) (2010) *Mental Health and Development: Targeting People with Mental Health Conditions as a Vulnerable Group*. Geneva: WHO.

Zigmond, A.S. and Snaith, R.D. (1983) The Hospital Anxiety and Depression Scale, *Acta Psychiatrica Scandinavica*, 67: 361–70.

5 Psychological interventions in the personality disorders

Denise Aspinall

Chapter aim and objectives

Aim

- To explore the conceptual basis of the term personality disorder, including proposed causes and interventions.

Objectives

- To identify personality disorder in terms of theories and in terms of classification.
- To describe and critique the evidence base underpinning the care of individuals with a personality disorder.
- To describe and apply psychological interventions that will promote a positive pathway in the care of individuals with a personality disorder.

What is a personality disorder?

Personality disorders as a diagnostic class are complex and controversial, indeed the concept itself and the need for a distinct disorder continue to be contested (O'Donohue et al., 2007; Castillo, 2009; Bennett, 2011). According to Winship and Hardy (2007: 148) 'personality disorder is the most prevalent psychiatric disorder' yet those diagnosed with a personality disorder are often perceived by the health-care professional to be either untreatable or difficult to manage. The data suggest that prevalence rates for personality disorders among adults living in the community are between 10 and 14 per cent (NIMHE, 2003a; Winship and Hardy, 2007). Jarrett (2006) reports that among psychiatric outpatients and in-patients this rises to between 30 and 40 per cent and 40 and 50 per cent respectively. Alwin et al. (2006: 1) state that 'between 50 per cent and 78 per cent of adult prisoners are believed to meet criteria for one or more personality disorder'.

As a student nurse you will work in various clinical areas and you will also be involved in the care of those diagnosed with a personality disorder. These clients will often be challenging and can be physically and emotionally draining on the resources of the team. Questions you may ask: why the individual may behave in a specific manner; the possible causative factors and theories; what interventions are available;

what works and what doesn't work? Hopefully by reading this chapter you may be able to understand the behaviour of your client and develop appropriate treatment strategies (DH, 2006a; 2006b; NMC, 2010).

After discussing what a personality disorder is, this chapter will focus primarily upon the diagnosis of borderline personality disorder. It is the most frequent personality disorder of those presenting to mental health services and more frequently diagnosed in women (Davey, 2008).

First let us look at how personality disorders are conceptualized, a good starting place is to explore what a personality is.

Davey (2008: 392) describes the term personalities as 'enduring features of individuals that determine how we respond to life events and experiences... providing a convenient means by which others can label and react to us'. Said to be relatively enduring, our personality is individual to us and our experiences but it is shaped by both our environment and psychological experiences, and uniquely influences our cognitions, motivations and behaviours in various situations. We all have our own ways of behaving and relating to others; that is what makes us unique!

Gordon Allport (1937) described two major ways to study personality: the nomothetic and the idiographic. The idiographic approach is concerned with the uniqueness of the individual, provides a rich and multifaceted description, and personal attributes and behaviour are investigated via case studies. The nomothetic approach is based on universal laws, has set parameters, looks at traits and is investigated via personality tests, meaning that individuals are compared in terms of a specific number of traits or dimensions common to everyone.

Gross (2010: 663) suggests that a definition of personality would be 'those relatively stable and enduring aspects of individuals which distinguish them from other people, making them unique, but which at the same time allow people to be compared to each other'. Personality traits describe 'regularities or consistencies of actions, thoughts or feelings – average behaviour over many settings and occasions' (Alwin et al., 2006: 5). The view that we all share the same personality features (traits), and that they can be registered on a continuum, is the basis of dimensional models of personality disorder.

Personality disorders are psychiatric conditions described in the two main classification systems – the *Diagnostic and Statistical Manual of Mental Disorders IV* (DSM-IV) (American Psychiatric Association (APA), 1994) and the *International Classification of Diseases 10* (ICD-10) (World Health Organization, 1992). The DSM-IV classification of personality disorder is based upon the concept of personality traits. Personality disorders are in a category of their own in the DSM-IV (APA, 1994) within Axis II, and are described as: 'An enduring pattern of inner experience and behaviour that deviates markedly from the expectations of the individual's culture, is pervasive and inflexible, has an onset in adolescence or early adulthood, is stable over time, and leads to distress or impairment' (APA, 1994: 629).

The ICD-10 defines a personality disorder as:

> [d]eeply ingrained and enduring behaviour patterns... they represent either extreme or significant deviations from the way the average individual in a given culture perceives, thinks, feels and particularly relates to others. Such

behaviour patterns tend to be stable and to encompass multiple domains of behaviour and psychological functioning. They are frequently, but not always, associated with various degrees of subjective distress and problems in social functioning and performance.

(World Health Organization, 1992: 200)

Borderline personality disorder is described as a 'pervasive pattern of instability of interpersonal relationships, self-image and affect, and marked impulsivity beginning by early adulthood and present in a variety of contexts' (APA, 2000).

Table 5.1 is adapted from the work of McMurran (2008: 377); it illustrates how the two classification systems compare and some of the traits or characteristics associated with each personality type. As you will see the DSM-IV 'clusters' the different personality disorders where the ICD-10 uses 'types', and for some diagnoses in the DSM-IV there are no equivalents in the ICD-10.

However O'Donohue et al. (2007) suggest that the terms and phrases used in the DSM-IV (APA, 1994) definition of personality disorder require further explanation;

Table 5.1 Comparing personality disorders (DSM-IV and ICD-10)

DSM-IV	ICD-10
Cluster A – Odd/eccentric personality disorder	*Types of disorder*
• Paranoid – suspiciousness	• Equivalent
• Schizoid – socially and emotionally detached	• Equivalent
• Schizotypal – social and interpersonal deficits	• No equivalent
Cluster B – Dramatic/emotional personality disorder	*Types of disorder*
• Antisocial – violation of the rights of others	• Dissocial – callous disregard of others, irresponsibility, irritability
• Borderline – instability of relationships, self-image and mood	• Emotionally unstable. Impulsive type – inability to control anger, unpredictable, quarrelsome. Borderline type – unclear self-image, intense, unstable relationships
• Histrionic – excessively emotional and attention-seeking	• Equivalent
• Narcissistic – grandiose, lack of empathy, need for admiration	• No equivalent
Cluster C – Anxious/fearful personality disorder	*Types of disorder*
• Avoidant – socially inhibited, feelings of inadequacy, hypersensitivity	• Equivalent
• Dependent – clinging, submissive	• Equivalent
• Obsessive compulsive – perfectionist, inflexible	• Anankastic – indecisive, pedantic, rigid

what does 'enduring' mean? If the term 'pattern' is an essential characteristic in the diagnosis of personality disorder, then how consistent has this pattern to be?

In terms of causation Davey (2008: 411) suggests: 'There is certainly no overarching or all-inclusive theory of the aetiology of personality disorders because the different clusters represent quite different patterns of behaviour, so we might expect that different clusters, and indeed, different personality disorders, may be acquired in quite different ways.'

Those diagnosed with borderline personality disorder are more likely than the general population to have been neglected and experienced separation from their parents (Bennett, 2011). Many of those diagnosed with borderline personality disorder will have experienced some form of trauma in childhood including physical and sexual abuse, violence and higher levels of childhood illness (Fossey and Black, 2010).

The notion of a personality disorder is not always viewed in terms of the medical model; psychological models also play a part. As an example, the psychoanalytic model tends to view personality disorders in terms of motivations and transference patterns, whereas the interpersonal model takes the view that personality disorders are related to an individual's early social learning (Davey, 2008).

To summarize this section the following scenario provides an illustrative example within the mental health-care field of the general impact a personality disorder can have upon the individual; we will look at this scenario in more detail in the psychological interventions section.

SCENARIO

Mary, a 20-year-old at the time of her admission, has been an in-patient on an acute mental health ward for the past 18 months. Mary's original diagnosis on admission was moderate-to-severe depression; she has since been diagnosed with a borderline personality disorder. The circumstances leading up to Mary's admission relate to Mary taking 40 paracetamol tablets with the clear intention of killing herself (as expressed by Mary on interview) and ending what Mary calls her 'suffering and despair'. Mary was found by chance by her mother after taking the overdose and, despite the seriousness of this incident, both Mary and her parents reluctantly accepted Mary's admission to a mental health ward. The aim of the admission was to assess Mary and to try to understand why this almost spontaneous incident (overdose) happened and then formulate an appropriate community care package.

Evidence-based practice

The treatment and management of individuals diagnosed with personality disorder has become a major issue that is of concern not only to mental health practitioners but also those working in criminal justice systems, primary care and social services (McMurran, 2008). It would seem that the concept of untreatability associated with those diagnosed with a personality disorder has previously dictated the services of-fered to this individual – if it can not be treated then is it realistic or feasible to offer treatment? Alwin et al. (2006: 52) suggest 'historically mental health services have not perceived treating people with such problems as part of their core services'.

The independent inquiry into the care and treatment of Michael Stone, diagnosed with a severe antisocial personality disorder, highlighted the difficulties in detaining and treating those diagnosed as untreatable. The amended 1983 Mental Health Act re-moved the emphasis upon 'treatability' for compulsory detention. The Act now allows compulsory detention provided an individual meets the criteria for detention even if they have an untreatable disorder (such as personality disorder?). Further, the require-ment to address risk even if the presenting disorder is not directly treated suggests that those presenting with a personality disorder can be detained and, if required, should be given a treatment plan (McMurran, 2008).

In 2003 the NIMHE reported that 'people with a primary diagnosis of personality disorder are frequently unable to access the care they need from secondary mental health services. A few Trusts have dedicated personality disorder services but these are the exception rather than the rule' (NIMHE, 2003a: 5). Emphasis was placed on reducing exclusion, risk and negative pathways of care, and the development of in-clusive, appropriate and supportive services. The NIMHE (2003b) outlined the skills, training and leadership required to develop and deliver new services for those diag-nosed with a personality disorder. The emphasis for mental health services was that no longer would there be any excuse *not* to treat this group of people. The NIMHE (2003a: 23) highlighted 'a range of treatment interventions are available for personality disor-der . . . there is a growing body of literature available on the efficacy of varying treatment approaches . . . there are real grounds for optimism that therapeutic interventions can work for personality disordered patients'.

Evidence-based practice can be defined as 'the use of best clinical evidence in making patient care decisions' (Polit and Beck, 2008: 3). In other words, as a nurse you use the best available evidence to guide and enhance your practice (see also the introductory chapter). In relation to individuals diagnosed with a personality disorder: 'The assessment process offers the opportunity to begin establishing the conditions for treatment by building credibility, forging positive expectations about treatment, beginning to establish a working relationship, and preparing the patient for therapy' (Livesley, 2003: 117).

Risk cannot be eliminated but it can be reduced or minimized and effectively managed if it has been clearly identified, 'risk assessment and management remains at the heart of mental health care' (Eales, 2009: 164), 'all mental health nurses should be able to comprehensively assess and respond to service users' individual needs and identified risks' (DH, 2006a: 30; 2006b) (see also Chapter 1). Up to 10 per cent of those diagnosed with borderline personality disorder commit suicide (Lieb et al., 2004), and more than 70 per cent had a history of attempted suicide in Soloff et al.'s study (2002). In addition there is a strong tendency towards self-harm, suicidal ideation and impulsive aggressive behaviour among this group (National Institute for Health and Clinical Excellence (NICE), 2009): 'emotional dysregulation, increasing emotional arousal reduces coping, leading to impulsive actions' (Livesley, 2003: 138).

The three main areas of risk that nurses would be interested in are self-harming, suicide and violence. For each of these risk factors sensitive questioning should be used if the risks are immediate or long term.

History taking should include questions about family relationships, and the individual's reactions to key developmental events and changes. 'Maltreatment and attachment problems are common in the BPD population' (Cartwright, 2006: 439). Has the client experienced any significant loss or incidents of trauma and deprivation? Was support forthcoming? As already discussed, the client with a borderline personality disorder is more likely to have experienced either or both. Peer relationships and important memories should be explored – does the individual's perception differ from that of others?

Focusing the assessment further, we would ask the client to describe themselves: 'It would be helpful if you tell me a little more about yourself, who are you, what sort of person are you?' Those with a borderline personality disorder will display a marked unstable sense of self; this is often a difficult task as most clients rarely access knowledge about themselves in this way. A discussion of interpersonal relations is likely to provide evidence of highly intense and unstable relationships (Cartwright, 2006). Social functioning is likely to be impaired, particularly if a co-morbid disorder is present. Is the client using adaptive/maladaptive coping mechanisms, for example cutting behaviour? In what way is this behaviour helping? An important aspect of any interview according to Livesley (2003) is to establish if there are any maladaptive thinking and interpersonal behaviour patterns; core schema can be revealed during other parts of the assessment; for example, when discussing how the individual copes with loss and separation.

Perceptual-cognitive symptoms are common in borderline personality disorder, and individuals with a borderline personality disorder will often describe themselves as experiencing amnesic episodes and detachment from what is going on around them. This may or may not relate to a physical cause but, even so, any neuropsychological symptoms such as any head injury should be explored further (Livesley, 2003).

The information gained during the assessment(s) should be used for a purpose; the client also needs to be assessed for their ability to engage in a psychological approach to treatment. If the client does not have the capacity to understand psychological explanations for their behaviour they are less likely to benefit (Livesley, 2003).

Roth and Fonagy (1998) suggest that those who are psychologically minded with low impulsivity are likely to benefit from psychological therapy. The NICE guidelines (2009) also suggests the following may be of benefit to those with a borderline personality disorder.

> *Cognitive analytical therapy (CAT)* Is based on the notion that a set of partially disso-
> ciated 'self-states' account for the features of borderline personality disorder;
> switching between these states results in dyscontrol of emotions including
> intense expression, impaired ability to self-reflect and depersonalization. CAT
> helps the client understand how 'harsh, problematic and punitive relationship
> patterns have been learned and continue to be re-enacted', and to learn new
> patterns of relating to oneself and others (NICE, 2009: 127).

Cognitive behavioural therapy (CBT) Focuses upon modifying dysfunctional emotional and cognitive responses to events through altering underlying beliefs rather than symptoms (Alwin et al., 2006). Treatment includes homework and testing of core beliefs and structures. 'There is evidence that the addition of CBT to usual treatment has benefit in terms of reducing the volume of suicidal acts, reducing dysfunctional beliefs and psychiatric symptom distress' (Davidson et al., 2006: 464).

Dialectic behavioural therapy (DBT) A mixture of cognitive behavioural therapy (CBT) and Zen practice, DBT addresses emotional vulnerability and deficits in the capacity/motivation to regulate inner experiences (Swales and Heard, 2010). DBT helps those diagnosed with borderline personality disorder to 'regulate their emotions by overcoming suffering through acceptance' (Johnson et al., 2010: 24). Individual and skills training groups are offered weekly for approximately a year.

The initial focus of this therapy is directed at reducing self-harm (Linehan, 1993). Once this is achieved, the therapy moves to developing emotional control skills and master mindfulness, interpersonal effectiveness, and increasing distress tolerance and emotional regulation (Johnson et al., 2010). Recent control trials show DBT to be effective in reducing self-harming behaviour and borderline personality disorder symptoms (Feigenbaum, 2007; McMain et al., 2009).

Other therapies A mentalization-based therapy; borderline personality disorder is understood to be 'a disorder of self result from developmental disturbance of attachment' leading to a failure to understand one's own mental state and that of others. The therapy aims to increase self-reflective capacity and includes both individual and group work (NICE, 2009: 153).

Therapeutic community treatments Intensive psychosocial treatment but the main focus is the therapeutic environment itself as the main agent of change. External control is kept to a minimum: members take a significant role in decision making and the everyday running of the unit (NIMHE, 2003a; NICE, 2009).

Medication The focus is on controlling symptoms rather than treating the personality disorder and, although medication can be used to alleviate symptoms of co-morbid conditions, it should not be used specifically for this condition (NICE, 2009).

Psychological interventions and scenario

In principle when working with individuals diagnosed with a personality disorder, a psychological therapy should be offered for not less than three months and all therapy should:

- be well structured
- work on adherence
- have a clear focus
- be coherent to all parties
- be long term

- be integrated with other services
- be a therapeutic partnership (Bateman and Tyrer, 2002; NICE, 2009).

These therapies should also be underpinned by the following therapeutic strategies.

- Build and maintain a collaborative relationship based upon hope, respect, understanding and acceptance of the client's problems.
- Maintain a consistent approach – the therapist sets limits and is able to recognize and show understanding of why a client may be trying to alter the 'frame of therapy'.
- Establish and maintain a 'valid' intervention process – the therapist validates the description given of the client's experience.
- Build and maintain motivation for change – often the most neglected, yet motivation for change should be checked regularly (Livesley, 2005).

It has to be acknowledged that in some cases a service user may have to travel through a number of therapeutic stages which have specific interventions (Livesley, 2005) before they are ready to engage in a appropriate therapy:

- *safety* – interventions to ensure safety of self and others; in an in-patient setting this may require increased observations; in the community an assertive outreach approach should be used with increased contact and support
- *containment* – interventions (general therapeutic strategies) to contain emotional and behavioural instability (includes medication) – keeping safe through controlling the present symptoms of distress
- *control and regulation* – interventions to reduce symptoms, promote self-control and management of emotions and impulses (psychological and/or medication) – starting therapy
- *exploration and change* – interventions to change the underlying factors, emotional, cognitive and situational, that contribute to the 'problem behaviour' – interventions
- *integration* – interventions that are focused on developing a more adaptive self – person changes (Livesley, 2005).

We will now look at how this staged approach relates to the chapter scenario in more detail.

SCENARIO

After speaking about the circumstances leading up to the overdose Mary became increasingly tearful and distressed, and subsequently started to demand to go home. After a long discussion it was decided that Mary could go on leave for a few days. The next day the ward staff received a phone call that Mary was being brought back to the ward by her family because they were unable to cope with her angry and distressed behaviour. On arrival Mary started verbally abusing her parents saying that they had betrayed her and she subsequently physically attacked her mother. The staff calmed the situation down diverting Mary away from her parents into a side-room. Mary's mum was quite distressed by the situation and felt that Mary's behaviour was symptomatic of Mary being 'ill'; she knew that Mary had a bad temper but she had not known her to attack people before – to Mary's mum and dad 'this behaviour was out of character'.

Two weeks into Mary's admission and a week prior to discharge, Mary took another overdose after buying paracetamol from the local chemist. Stating her intention was to die, Mary changed her mind because she did not want to get the staff in trouble and therefore confided to a staff member what she had done. Mary then disclosed that she had also started to cut herself; a former patient on the ward had taught Mary how to self-harm in way which she believed relieved her 'despair'.

Eighteen months later Mary is still in hospital as the multidisciplinary team find it difficult to discharge her. Mary's self-harming behaviour escalates when discharge is planned or even talked about. Usually Mary will concentrate on cutting her arms or legs and has become so expert in cutting herself that she can control blood loss through the 'packing' of her wounds with paper. Mary can be quite impulsive with both her 'cutting behaviour' and her 'bouts of anger' if she feels her 'favourite' staff are not being 'responsive to her needs' or if staff are 'too challenging'. Mary is currently awaiting transfer to a therapeutic community but only if she demonstrates that she is willing to change her behaviour (admission criteria).

What can you see emerging from this scenario considering the staged approach?

In relation to this scenario in the early stages Mary's safety was the primary concern, hence her admission. A full multidisciplinary assessment was conducted and a risk management plan implemented with Mary's agreement and her family's knowledge. Mary was placed on one-to-one observations until any future risk of taking a further overdose was reduced. De-escalation techniques were frequently used to reduce the aggressive outbursts Mary presented with and, post-incident, all staff members were encouraged to discuss the reasons for her behaviour with Mary. Validation of Mary's distress was important in developing a therapeutic relationship (Linehan, 1993). In order to prepare her for more formal therapy Mary was encouraged to change her behaviour through motivational work during time set aside with a nurse therapist. As Mary had started to build good relationships with certain members of the nursing staff on the ward it was decided to use these relationships to help Mary control her self-harming behaviour. The focal part of this relationship building was agreed with Mary and Mary's psychiatrist to start sessional work around controlling self-harming behaviour. The long-term goal was for Mary to engage in dialectic behavioural therapy. Unfortunately she decided not to engage with this.

Mary described symptoms of depression, feeling low and in despair with little hope for the future. Mary was prescribed antidepressants for this. As Mary's behaviour became more settled, problem solving (CBT) and problem solving techniques, especially in relation to feeling 'depressed', were offered to her. These were targeted towards anger management, helping her to explore and encourage healthy expressions of anger, teaching her self-responsibility and exploring alternatives for destructive behaviour. Often those diagnosed with a borderline personality disorder have little sense of boundaries (Livesley, 2003).

While on the ward Mary was encouraged to use a daily journal, to help guide her to explore her feelings and interpersonal work focused on increasing her coping strategies when distressed. The ward staff were supported through supervision, particularly during high stress periods when Mary repeatedly self-harmed. NICE (2009) guidelines state quite clearly that clients like Mary should be cared for in the community and referrals were made to her local Community Mental Health Team prior to each proposed discharge date. As stated above Mary is no longer high risk although she remains impulsive and is now awaiting a place in a therapeutic community. Hospitalization for Mary has proved unhelpful and it is hoped that by being challenged about her maladaptive behaviour by others living in a therapeutic community she will learn more appropriate methods of coping with anger, distress and attachment issues. 'People with personality disorder can behave in ways that invite rejection . . . Skills and knowledge are required to enable staff to understand the reasons for this behaviour' (NIMHE, 2003b: 11).

Often services have responded ad hoc and usually reactively when a person has self-harmed or presents in crisis, the individual is then offered inappropriate admissions with little structured follow-up and those with a personality disorder report negativity, hostility and disrespect when they have presented to services (NIMHE, 2003a; 2003b).

Some four years after this statement was made, mental health nurses' attitudes were still found to be negative and less than favourable towards this client group, particularly towards those with a diagnosis of borderline personality disorder admitted to in-patient settings (Bland et al., 2007; James and Cowman, 2007). Yet clients rate trust as an essential component of the therapeutic relationship, without which a successful intervention was deemed to be unlikely (Langley and Klopper, 2005). Self-harming behaviour is viewed as attention seeking, and this was certainly the case with Mary initially, yet the reasons behind it are often complex and difficulty in self-regulation can lead to aggression and subsequent conflict with health-care professionals (Eastwick and Grant, 2005). Understanding of the reasons behind the behaviour would seem a logical step and would aid caregivers in the management of this client group. Those diagnosed with a borderline personality disorder have sometimes been excluded from services because care staff may lack confidence in their skill to manage this group of individuals, but it is promising to observe that since 2003 there has been an increase in training provision for health-care professionals. In our scenario staff would be encouraged to express their feelings and frustrations in supportive clinical supervision sessions, thus improving the quality of the care delivered to Mary.

Summary of the key points

Mental health nurses should actively seek to form a therapeutic relationship with their client, recognizing the need for the client's involvement in their care.

Mental health nurses should use a validating approach, recognizing that maladaptive behaviour is directly linked to past experience and the distress experienced by the client is very real to them.

Mental health nurses have to consider that working with this client group can be frustrating and challenging. Robust supervision, consistent team working and an understanding of why clients may behave in a specific manner should be sought.

Mental health nurses have to practise in a non-judgemental and holistic manner to provide an appropriate and positive care pathway for this client group.

Quick quiz

1 The *Diagnostic Statistical Manual IV* officially recognizes how many personality disorders?
2 In which axis is personality disorder assigned?
3 How are the individual diagnoses organized?
4 How many groups are there?
5 Name three of the recognized personality disorders?
6 Borderline personality disorder – give three characteristics.
7 Name two interventions for people with personality disorder?
8 Name a pivotal document in the development of services for those with a personality disorder?

References

Allport, G.W. (1937) Personality: a psychological interpretation, in W.J. Livesley (ed.) *Practical Management of Personality Disorder*. New York: Guilford Press.

Alwin, N., Blackburn, R., Davidson, K., Hilton, M., Logan, C. and Shine, J. (2006) *Understanding Personality Disorder: A Report by the British Psychological Society*. Leicester: British Psychological Society.

American Psychiatric Association (APA) (1994) *Diagnostic and Statistical Manual of Mental Disorders*. Washington, DC: APA.

American Psychiatric Association (APA) (2000) *Diagnostic and Statistical Manual of Mental Disorders*. 4th edn text revision (DSM–IV-TR). Washington, DC: APA.

Bateman, A. and Tyrer, P. (2002) Effective management of personality disorder, in National Institute for Mental Health in England (2003a) *Personality Disorder: No Longer a Diagnosis of Exclusion. Policy Implementation Guidance for the Development of Services for People with Personality Disorder*. London: NIMHE.

Bennett, P. (2011) *Abnormal and Clinical Psychology: An Introductory Textbook*, 3rd edn. Maidenhead: McGraw-Hill.

Bland, A.R., Tudor, G. and Whitehouse, D.M. (2007) Nursing care of inpatients with borderline personality disorder, *Perspectives in Psychiatric Care*, 43(4): 204–12.

Cartwright, D. (2006) Borderline personality disorder: what do we know? Diagnosis, course, co-morbidity, and aetiology, *South African Journal of Psychology*, 38(2): 429–46.

Castillo, H. (2009) The person with a personality disorder, in I. Norman and I. Ryrie (eds) *The Art and Science of Mental Health Nursing: A Textbook of Principles and Practice*, 2nd edn. Maidenhead: McGraw-Hill.

Davey, G. (2008) *Psychopathology: Research, Assessment and Treatment in Clinical Psychology.* Leicester: British Psychological Society and Blackwell Publishing.

Davidson, K., Norrie, J., Tyrer, P., Gumley, A., Tata, P., Murray, H. and Palmer, S. (2006) The effectiveness of cognitive behavior therapy for borderline personality disorder: results from the Borderline Personality Disorder Study of Cognitive Therapy (Boscot) trial, *Journal of Personality Disorders,* 20(5): 450–65.

Department of Health (DH) (2006a) *From Values to Action: The Chief Nursing Officer's Review of Mental Health Nursing.* London: Department of Health.

Department of Health (DH) (2006b) *Best Practice Competencies and Capabilities for Pre-registration Mental Health Nurses in England: The Chief Nursing Officer's Review of Mental Health Nursing.* London: Department of Health.

Eales, S. (2009) Risk assessment and management, in P. Callaghan, J. Playle and L. Cooper (eds) *Mental Health Nursing Skills.* Oxford: Oxford University Press.

Eastwick, Z. and Grant, A. (2005) The treatment of people with borderline personality disorder: a cause for concern? *Mental Health Practice,* 8(7): 38–40.

Feigenbaum, J. (2007) Dialectical behaviour therapy: an increasing evidence base, *Journal of Mental Health,* 16(1): 51–68.

Fossey, M. and Black, G. (2010) *Under the Radar, Women with Borderline Personality Disorder in Prison.* London: Centre for Mental Health.

Gross, R. (2010) *Psychology: The Science of Mind and Behaviour,* 6th edn. London: Hodder.

James, P.D. and Cowman, S. (2007) Psychiatric nurses' knowledge, experience and attitudes towards clients with borderline personality disorder, *Journal of Psychiatric and Mental Health Nursing,* 14(7): 670–8.

Jarrett, C. (2006) Understanding personality disorder, *The Psychologist,* 19(7): 402–4.

Johnson, A.B., Gentile, J.P. and Correll, T.L. (2010) Accurately diagnosing and treating borderline personality disorder: a psychotherapeutic case. *Psychiatry (Edgemont),* 7(4): 21–30.

Langley, G. and Klopper, H. (2005) Trust as a therapeutic foundation for patients with borderline personality disorder, *Journal of Psychiatric and Mental Health Nursing,* 12(1): 23–32.

Lieb, K., Zanarini, M.C., Schmahl, C., Linehan, M.M. and Bohus, M. (2004) Borderline personality disorder, *Lancet,* 364: 453–61.

Linehan, M.M. (1993) *Skills Training Manual for Treating Personality Disorder.* New York: Guilford Press.

Livesley, W.J. (2003) *Practical Management of Personality Disorder.* New York: Guilford Press.

Livesley, W.J. (2005) Principles and strategies for treating personality disorder, *Canadian Journal of Psychiatry,* 50(8): 442–50.

McMain, S.F., Links, P.S., Gnam, W.H., Guimond, T., Cardish, R.J., Kormann, L. and Streiner, D.I. (2009) A randomised controlled trial of dialectical behaviour therapy versus general psychiatric management for borderline personality disorder, *American Journal of Psychiatry,* 166(12): 1365–74.

McMurran, M. (2008) Personality disorders, in K. Soothill, P. Rogers and M. Dolan (eds) *Handbook of Forensic Mental Health.* Cullompton: Willan.

National Institute for Clinical Excellence (NICE) (2009) *Borderline Personality Disorder.* London: NICE.

National Institute for Mental Health in England (NIMHE) (2003a) *Personality Disorder: No Longer a Diagnosis of Exclusion. Policy Implementation Guidance for the Development of Services for People with Personality Disorder*. London: NIMHE.

National Institute for Mental Health in England (NIMHE) (2003b) *Breaking the Cycle of Rejection: The Personality Disorder Capabilities Framework*. London: NIMHE.

Nursing and Midwifery Council (2010) *Standards for Pre-registration Nursing Education*. London: Nursing and Midwifery Council.

O'Donohue, W., Fowler, K. and Lilienfeld, S. (2007) *Personality Disorders: Towards the DSM-V*. London: Sage.

Polit, D.F. and Beck, C.T. (2008) *Nursing Research: Generating and Accessing Evidence for Nursing Practice*, 8th edn. London: Lippincott, Williams and Wilkins.

Roth, A. and Fonaghy, P. (1998) What works for whom? A critical review of psychotherapy research, in P. Bennett (2011) *Abnormal and Clinical Psychology: An Introductory Textbook*, 3rd edn. Maidenhead: McGraw-Hill.

Soloff, P.H., Lynch, K.G. and Kelly, T.M. (2002) Childhood abuse as a risk factor for suicidal behaviour in borderline personality disorder, in A.L. Holm and E. Severinsson (eds) The emotional pain and distress of borderline personality disorder: a review of the literature, *International Journal of Mental Health Nursing*, 17: 27–35.

Swales, M.A. and Heard, H.L. (2010) *Dialectical Behavioral Therapy*. New York: Routledge.

Winship, G. and Hardy, S. (2007) Perspectives on the prevalence and treatment of personality disorder, *Journal of Psychiatric and Mental Health Nursing*, 14(2): 148–54.

World Health Organization (1992) *International Classification of Diseases 10*. Geneva: WHO.

6 Psychological interventions in drugs and alcohol

May Baker

Chapter aim and objectives

Aim

- To explore drugs and alcohol within a contemporary mental health nursing context.

Objectives

- To distinguish between drug effects and their legal classification.
- To identify the relevant evidence-based practice and policy.
- To describe, analyse and apply psychological interventions within a drugs and alcohol context.

An introduction to drug and alcohol dependency

This chapter will discuss drug and alcohol use within society and the issues this may pose for contemporary mental health nursing. It will further explore evidence-based practice and policy, and discuss psychological interventions used to overcome drug and alcohol problems. This chapter will not be able to describe or discuss in detail every drug available; however, this chapter will endeavour to distinguish between drug effects and their legal classification.

Alcohol is consumed by half of the world's population and is one of the most widely used drugs. In England alone 90 per cent of the adult population drink alcohol, with 24 per cent drinking in a harmful way and 4 per cent dependent (NICE, 2011). The alcohol needs assessment research project (DH, 2004) found that 7.1 million people in England are drinking at harmful levels. In comparison the estimated prevalence of problematic opiate use (heroin) in England is 273,123, with the British Crime Survey (2009) reporting that problematic opiate use was rare within the general household population, at 0.1 per cent. However, cannabis is by far the most widely used illicit drug in the world. Between 143 and 190 million people reported using cannabis at least once in 2007 (UNODC, 2009). It is the most frequently used illicit drug in the UK, with 3.5 million users.

Before examining the broader picture of drug and alcohol use it would be prudent to briefly examine the terminology used for drug and alcohol use, which at times can be detrimental and hinder the therapeutic relationship between the user and the nurse, further damaging the process of any productive psychological intervention. Alcohol abuse and drug addict are common sayings, but what is meant by these terms and do they give a fair picture of the individuals who use these substances?

As professionals we should encourage and use language that de-stigmatizes those individuals who misuse drugs. Finding different words or phrases that are less value laden can help a person acknowledge and seek help for their problem (Barker and Buchanan-Barker, 2009). If that person views the professional as someone who judges by using terms such as 'alcoholic' or 'heroin addict' then they may decide not to engage with services and therefore the opportunity to help could be lost. Therefore, how can the word 'misusing' be explained within the context of drug and alcohol use? If we misuse a pen, for instance, we are using it wrongly, perhaps by trying to write with it from the other end. However if we misuse alcohol or drugs how do we know this? What is the benchmark and how is this measured?

The Department of Health (DH, 2007) provides guidance on sensible limits for those who drink alcohol and offers a marker for comparison. This relates to levels that would have the least detrimental effects on health (Kipping, 2004) (see Box 5.1). However it is a somewhat different picture when reflecting on drug use. First, street drugs are illegal and therefore the monitoring and measurement of such use is difficult to obtain. There are agencies who manage to do this with a degree of validity (EMCDDA, 2009; UNODC, 2009) but measuring how much of a drug an individual uses can be hit and miss. This may be because the illicit drug passes along several people before eventually being sold to the person who will use it. As the drug moves through the line of 'dealers' it can be adulterated with bulking agents such as talcum powder or caffeine to enable the drug dealer to get the maximum return on their drug, easily making a 1 kg weight become 2 kg. The process of adulteration can cause physical problems for some users who inject, by causing blocked veins, pulmonary embolisms, thrombosis and abscesses (Wilson, 2011).

Prescribed drugs and over-the-counter medicines are dispensed legally by pharmacists but they too can be misused. Although they are not adulterated they are often sold on the 'black market' to people for whom they were not prescribed. Therefore, trying to measure how much a person uses is not straightforward and can depend largely on whose measurement criteria we adopt. This can be difficult as the ingredients for illicit drugs can change from place to place and dealer to dealer, however alcohol, as a legal drug, is licensed for consumption and therefore monitored prior to being sold to the public.

It is important to also note how society views illicit drug use. Some drugs, although illegal, are much more accepted in society. Within any social circle illegal drugs may be placed within an order of acceptability: some groups may deem cannabis fully acceptable while others may condone the use of cocaine and amphetamine for recreational use. Many groups would condemn the use of heroin, which the media portrays in an extremely negative way (Marsden et al., 2004). Therefore the attitude, knowledge and skills the nurse holds is paramount when engaging the person in the care process.

Box 5.1 Alcohol consumption table

Formula for calculating alcohol units

$$\frac{\text{Alcohol by volume} \times \text{ml}}{1000}$$

8 g of ethanol = a standard drink (UK) = 1 unit =
25 ml spirits at 40% volume,
$\frac{1}{2}$ pint of lager at 3.5% volume, or
100 ml wine at 10% volume

Sensible guidelines for drinking

Women 2–3 units daily (14 units weekly)
Men 3–4 units daily (21 units weekly)
Weekly units should not be consumed all
    at once
2 days' abstinence is recommended
Binge drinking for women is >6 units and
    for men >8 units in any one session

Previous attitudinal studies found that nurses bore a negative attitude to substance misusers (Macloughlin and Long, 1996; Rassool, 1998; Sellick and Redding, 1998), however, recent studies by Rassool (2006; 2007) revealed that undergraduate nursing students held more positive attitudes to those with a pharmacological addiction. This could partly be due to the rise in the profile of substance misuse within education and training in nursing and medicine, which can only benefit service provision. Therefore, in defining drug use, terminology should not be 'loaded' in a way that is unhelpful in the therapeutic process and that of engaging the person in treatment.

The following descriptions may help you to clarify things:

Drug: a drug is any chemical agent that affects biologic function ... A psychoactive drug is one that acts in the brain to alter mood, thought processes or behaviour.

Drug use: the non-problematic use of drugs usually prescribed medication ... This use may still carry the potential for adverse effects. Drug use is socially acceptable whereas drug misuse and drug abuse tend to have negative connotations (Wilson, 2011: 364).

Drug misuse: this usually means that the person is using the drug in a socially unacceptable manner, which would normally be dictated by the culture or country to which they belong. The drug use also has a detrimental effect on their physical, social or psychological well-being.

Drug dependence: when someone has a compulsion to use a drug, for either the physical or psychological effects. The cessation of this drug can lead to withdrawal. The word addicted can also be used but some people see this as a negative term. See ICD-10 (WHO, 1994) for the criteria of drug dependence.

Alcohol is a legal drug, made from ethanol (Rassool, 2011). It suppresses the central nervous system, giving feelings of relaxation and mild stimulation. However, in larger doses alcohol will impair functioning and cognition and can lead to serious physical and mental health problems. The potential for harm is sometimes minimized as professionals may overlook or misinterpret signs and symptoms. Consumption is measured by standardized units (see Box 5.1). However, it should be noted that different countries will have different standardized units for recommended sensible guidelines for alcohol. Binge drinking (when a person consumes double the recommended units in one day) and hazardous drinking (when men consume 22–50 units weekly and women 15–35 weekly) and harmful drinking (men consume over 50 units weekly and women over 35 units weekly) are a major concern to health professionals who have to deal with the consequences of problematic alcohol use (DH, 2007).

There are many physical, psychological and social problems associated with heavy or binge drinking, which include poor concentration, irritability, depression, anxiety, panic attacks, sleep problems, paranoia and memory loss. There can also be severe long-term physical problems associated with heavy dependent drinking. These include diabetes, neuropathy, raised blood pressure, cancers, pancreatitis, foetal harm, Wernicke-Korsakoff psychosis and cirrhosis of the liver. The lack of social interaction and apathy through drinking can also impact on a person's mental health. Some problems associated with this type of drinking include relationship, debt, legal and work problems (Baker and Buckley, 2011).

Drugs, on the other hand, mainly refer to what is available on the illegal market. This can be confusing for some health professionals unless they work closely with or within drug services. It is often difficult to keep up with the changing climate as new drugs appear on the market. Drugs can ebb and flow with time and are linked intrinsically to availability, popular culture and, in some instances, to the music scene. There are also drugs which are known as 'legal highs', such as mephedrone which until recently could be purchased legally over the Internet until it was made illegal to do so.

Two ways in which drugs are classified are through their effect and their legality. This means the effect that the drug has on a person from a physical and psychological perspective, and the legal status of the drug (Wilson, 2011). The effect a drug has on a person can be classified as either stimulant, depressant or hallucinogenic. Different drugs have different effects on our central nervous system (CNS). For example, cocaine (upper) is a stimulant which increases activity within the CNS, causing arousal and restlessness, whereas opiates (downers) as depressants decrease activity within the CNS, causing drowsiness and reduced reflex functioning within the respiratory tract. Other drugs such as lysergic acid diethylamide (LSD) and psilocybin (magic mushrooms) are classed as hallucinogenic as they distort perception. Some drugs may be viewed as having two classifications, such as cannabis which may have mild hallucinogenic properties but also acts as a depressant on the CNS. It is not the purpose of this chapter to identify and describe every illicit drug, however for a comprehensive overview of the effects of drugs on the CNS please refer to FRANK (2011).

The legal classification of drugs relates to the law under the Misuse of Drugs Act 1971. The drugs subject to this Act are named as 'controlled' drugs. The Act lists three classes of controlled drugs. Those drugs thought to be most harmful are in Class A and those thought to be less harmful are in Classes B and C. It should be noted that the likelihood of death, injury, mental disturbance or drug dependence is not necessarily any less for users of Class C or Class B than it is for users of Class A. The penalties sustained if either caught dealing or using illicit drugs will depend largely on the drug's classification. Some commonly used drugs in Class A are heroin, cocaine and ecstasy;

in class B, cannabis, amphetamine and mephedrone; and in class C, benzodiazepine, gammahydroxybutyrate (GHB) and anabolic steroids. For further information on the illicit drug market please refer to FRANK (2011).

There is no firm explanation as to why people use drugs; there could be many reasons. Some evidence highlights stress, peer pressure, family disruption or to mask painful experiences such as neglect or abuse (Kumpfer and Bluth, 2004; Frischer et al. 2005; Prescott et al., 2006). People's drug use can change with time; some outgrow their drug use and stop. Others may experiment with different drugs or become dependent. At some point they may seek help and advice from services in dealing with their problem. Nurses will not just be treating people who are physically dependent on drugs or alcohol but will see the spectrum of drug and alcohol use throughout their working lives. Taking this into account, the following two scenarios provide illustrative examples of this. These examples will be explored further in the psychological interventions section.

DRUGS SCENARIO

Meg likes to use heroin, she needs it just to function. She always uses when Greg calls round and they 'cook up' together. Greg tries to pace himself when he uses but Meg loves getting smashed with him. She thinks she must spend £80 a day and never knows how she is going to afford it but something always turns up and she manages to scrape enough money together to get what she needs each day. This has been going on for a while now and Greg is worried that Meg is 'losing it'. He thinks she's been overdoing it but she doesn't seem to want to listen to him. She just keeps telling him this helps her forget and that she needs him.

ALCOHOL SCENARIO

Johnny is 45 years old and has been drinking heavily for 25 years. He is well known to alcohol services and has had several detoxes over the past 15 years. His longest period of abstinence has been two years; he states this was due to the birth of his son Joey who is now 10 years old. Following detoxification he remains abstinent by attending a 12-step programme which is held at his local community centre. He usually relapses quite quickly when he stops attending the programme and cuts himself off from his support system in Alcoholics Anonymous (AA).

Evidence-based practice

The importance of evidence-based practice and policy is explored in this section. The foundation for best practice has to come from available evidence. This means as professionals we should offer treatment that is in the patient's best interests and should be tailored to suit them. Consideration in availability and cost will at some point come into the equation, however, best practice can also be achieved using innovation and inventiveness. Policy relating to drug use is presently available in the government's 10-year strategy, Drugs: Protecting Families and Communities (HM Government, 2008). The four themes of this policy relate to: drug supply and crime; early intervention in relation to children, young people and families; a whole systems approach to drug treatment which encompasses agencies such as housing and employment; and, finally, public campaigns such as the national drug information campaign, which informs the public on the harm and risk of drug taking. Drug policy from Scotland, Wales and Northern Ireland, while having similarities, also relates to recovery, harm reduction, prevention, treatment, law and criminal justice.

In contrast, the policy relating to alcohol and tobacco has been controversial due to their legality and the revenue they make for the government through taxation. The policy, Safe, Sensible and Social (DH, 2007), focused on young people's drinking, which included binge drinking and those who drink at harmful levels but may not realize the potential for physical and mental health problems. The current government is reviewing this alcohol strategy with a focus on licensing, pricing, taxation and underage drinking (Alcohol Policy UK, 2010). However, both policies have at their forefront the themes of young people and health.

Several interventions can be used in the treatment of drug and alcohol use and it would be wise to mention pharmacology prior to discussing psychological interventions. Treating drug use solely with a psychological approach tends to be used with drugs where there is little or no evidence for the use of pharmacology, for instance cannabis and cocaine. Pharmacological (medication) intervention supported by psychological intervention is used with drugs where there is a physical addiction, such as opiates and alcohol. Therefore, pharmacology can help the person to stop using altogether (in the case of detoxification) or it may help to support the person once they have stopped (abstinence/relapse prevention). Best practice would suggest that pharmacological intervention should be used in conjunction with psychological interventions as better outcomes are achieved (NICE, 2011).

There are different types of medication used to control withdrawal and help maintain abstinence, some of which are listed below. Medication used for the cessation and abstinence of tobacco will not be discussed in this chapter.

The generic names are followed by the trade names in brackets. This list is not exhaustive and for further guidance on other medication and dosage please refer to NICE guidelines (2011) or BNF (2010).

Medication used in alcohol detoxification:
- Benzodiazepine (chlordiazepoxide or diazepam)
- Clomethiazole (Heminevrin) used for in patient setting only, as associated with a risk for dependence.

Medication used to prevent relapse in alcohol addiction:
- Disulfiram (Antabuse)
- Acamprosate (Campral EC).

Medication used for opiate detoxification:
- Methadone (also used for maintenance – see DH guidelines)
- Lofexedine (Britlofex)
- Buprenorphine (subutex).

Medication used to prevent relapse in opiate addiction:
- Naltrexone (nalorex).

There are many psychological interventions that can be used when addressing drug and alcohol problems, some of which can be used in both areas. This chapter will focus on the key psychological interventions that are endorsed by evidenced research and are widely used in contemporary practice.

NICE (2007; 2011) declares that psychological interventions in drug and alcohol problems should be tailored for the person. The National Treatment Agency (NTA) is a special health authority, created by the government in 2001, with a remit to increase the availability, capacity and effectiveness of treatment for drug misuse in England. It uses the models of care approach. This approach for both alcohol and drugs outlines the framework for providing and commissioning evidence-based treatment in England. Models of Care for Alcohol Misusers (MoCAM) and Models of Care for Drug Misusers (MoCDM) both offer structured treatment and integrated care pathways to suit the individual service user.

MoCAM and MoCDM work within a four-tier framework of service provision. Further information on this system is available via the NTA *Moa 's of Care* (2006; 2007). The psychological intervention offered will depend on the extent of the person's problem. Key interventions/therapies include:

- motivational enhancement therapy (MET)
- cognitive behavioural therapy (CBT), including couples therapy
- 12-step facilitation therapy
- social behaviour and network therapy
- coping and social skills training.

Sometimes combinations of therapies are used and the availability of these psychosocial therapies should be accessible for a wide range of the population, including those with complex and diverse needs. For the purpose of this chapter I will focus on two interventions.

Motivational enhancement therapy is a therapy which derives from 'motivational interviewing', a technique developed by Miller and Rollnick to resolve ambivalence and help the client change their behaviour. 'Motivational Interviewing is a client-centred directive method for enhancing intrinsic motivation to change, by exploring and resolving ambivalence' (Miller and Rollnick, 2002: 25).

This means that the therapist helps the person to clear up any dilemma they have about changing their behaviour. It helps to identify clearly that the person is resolving their problem and they are in control. The therapist works in a facilitating role which leads the person to their own conclusions and goals. There are five strategies used in MET, as listed below with an explanation of what they mean.

Express empathy by using reflective listening to convey understanding of the persons point of view and underlying drives.

Develop the discrepancy between the person's most deeply held values and their current behaviour (that is, tease out ways in which current unhealthy behaviours conflict with the wish to 'be good' – or to be viewed to be good).

Avoid arguing by not getting into an argument with the person, but *sidestep resistance* by responding with empathy and understanding rather than confrontation.

Support self-efficacy by building the person's confidence that change is possible.

Overall the therapist's aim is to support the person, encouraging them to be confident and to believe that they can change, meanwhile getting them to reflect on their behaviour and how that may conflict with their own deep values. Remember these values may be different to those of the nurse. The idea is *not* to argue or be confrontational with the person but to roll with their resistance through understanding and empathy.

The skills that a good motivational therapist needs are to:

- understand the other person's frame of reference
- filter the person's thoughts so that statements encouraging change are amplified and statements that reflect the status quo are dampened down
- elicit from the person statements that encourage change, such as expressions of problem recognition, concern, desire, intention to change
- match the process used in the theory to the stage of change; ensure that they do not jump ahead of the person
- express acceptance and affirmation
- affirm the person's freedom of choice and self-direction (adapted from Treasure, 2004).

In contrast the 12-step facilitation therapy has a different approach. Created by the self-help group Alcoholics Anonymous (AA), the interventions focus on self-help and support through a network of people who have also had drug or alcohol problems. AA was developed through the temperance movement in the 1930s and has a worldwide following. Further 12-step programmes such as Narcotics Anonymous and Al-Ateen follow the same principal. The basis of the 12 steps is for the individual to declare to others their addiction and state that they have no control over their compulsion to use the drug/alcohol, and call on the higher power of god to help them to recover from the temptation. The goal of the 12-step approach is total abstinence, and support is given also on a one-to-one level by a sponsor, a person who is also in recovery from their addiction (AA, 2011).

Psychological interventions and scenarios

Before examining the key interventions used for treating drug problems, the process of engaging the patient in a therapeutic meaningful relationship is paramount. This engagement supports and encourages them throughout their journey. The professional must help to engage the patient in treatment, and by doing so can then explore their anxieties, hopes and aspirations. The relationship between the patient and the professional can be a powerful source in achieving a positive outcome. The attitude of the professional nurse is vital in helping to keep the patient in treatment and helping them achieve their goal (Cooper, 2009; NICE, 2011)

By using a person-centred approach the patient is actively encouraged to engage with services for treatment of their drug problem. This approach advocates autonomy on the patient's part, ensuring their needs and wants are recognized and take centre stage when goals are planned. If the nurse is confrontational rather than supportive, then the patient is more likely to disengage with services. This can be likened to being served at your local grocery store. If the sales assistant is uninterested and unhelpful then you are more likely to leave and go to another shop where you will receive better service. Unfortunately, the patient may not have any choice in where they go for treatment, therefore it is imperative that staff who work in drug and alcohol services are not only competent in providing treatment, but are also skilled in engaging patients and promoting patient autonomy (NTA, 2006).

Prior to using any psychological intervention, the nurse should assess from a biopsychosocial perspective and include the following:

- What drug?
- How much, how often, how taken?
- Where taken?
- With whom?
- What triggers?
- What consequences?

Understanding how motivated a person is can be crucial in the drug and alcohol assessment. Imagine if the nurse suggests to the person she is assessing that they would benefit greatly from bereavement counselling. She has come to that conclusion as the person repeatedly states that they have never got over the death of their child and uses alcohol to cope. This may be the case, but at this stage the person may not be ready to undertake bereavement counselling. Finding out where a person is up to in their readiness to change will help the nurse to facilitate the recovery process without setting the person up to fail. It may be that the person is still drinking heavily and as yet has not contemplated giving up alcohol, and therefore would not yet be suitable for counselling.

A model to help in identifying readiness to change is Prochaska and DiClemente's (1986) model of change. They describe six stages of behaviour change, which work in a cyclical fashion:

1   pre-contemplation – not recognizing the problem
2   contemplation – recognition
3   action – doing something about it
4   making changes – attempting behaviour change
5   maintaining change – keeping this change going
6   relapse – returning to the original behaviour.

DRUGS SCENARIO

In relation to the drugs scenario, by trying to utilize MET the nurse may wish to consider how to engage Meg into treatment. She most probably is in the pre-contemplation part of the cycle of change, which means that she is not really thinking about her drug use and the impact it is having on her and others. The person who may seek out help for Meg is most probably Greg. He can encourage her to go to her GP who can then refer her on to the most appropriate service. During the assessment phase it is important for the nurse to be empathic and understanding, as this will give confidence to Meg and help her to open up and talk about her problem. The next step would be to tease out ways in which her current chaotic drug use conflicts with how she wishes to be perceived. Meanwhile, it is important for the nurse to avoid getting into any arguments with Meg and sidestep resistance with understanding rather than confrontation. Finally, in order to move forward, the nurse should try to instil self-efficacy and empowerment to Meg by offering non-judgemental support and hope for the future.

ALCOHOL SCENARIO

Referring to the alcohol scenario, Johnny has started drinking heavily again after a four-month period of abstinence. He has arrived at the clinic for an assessment of his needs with a view to detoxifying. He tells the nurse that he feels he knows all there is to know about 'booze' but just needs one more detox and he will 'never drink again' as his wife has had enough and has given him an ultimatum to stop drinking or leave the family home. He says he could never leave his son and wants to be a good dad, so this time he is going to do it.

The nurse is very concerned about Johnny's physical health as his blood results indicate that he now has severe liver damage. He looks jaundiced and appears un-dernourished and thin. Johnny is in the action stage of the cycle of change, as he is actively seeking help for his problem. However, the immediate priority is his physical health. He would need to be admitted to a medical ward for a full physical examination and treatment in relation to his health needs. Once his physical health is stable, or during this period, Johnny should be encouraged by the nurse to re-establish links with his 12-step sponsor. This approach has worked well for him in the past and, owing to his physical health problems, abstinence is the preferable option.

The nurse can act as facilitator in this process, encouraging him to make contact with the service/sponsor. She may also help him to locate the nearest 12-step meeting place and arrange transport for him if needed. The nurse should emphasize the importance of remaining abstinent not only because of his chronic health problem but also because of his family. The nurse should approach this in an empathic way while trying to empower Johnny in the choices that he has made.

Summary of the key points

The vast majority of people do not have problems associated with drugs and alcohol; however, for those who do, service provision and treatment should reflect their needs, taking into account culture, gender and diversity.

The nurse who is involved with people who misuse drugs and alcohol has to have a working knowledge of this area while utilizing their skills to promote awareness within their profession.

Psychological interventions are part and parcel of drug and alcohol treatment, and the use of such therapies should not be underestimated.

Pharmacological therapy alone is not sufficient for the complexities of drug and alcohol problems.

Quick quiz

1   What is one of the most widely used drugs in the world?
2   Why is it difficult to measure the amount of heroin a drug user may take?
3   What is the difference between drug use, misuse and dependence?
4   What are the weekly sensible alcohol limits for men and women?
5   Name three psychological and three physical problems associated with heavy alcohol use?
6   Name two ways in which drugs are classified?
7   Why do people use drugs?
8   Name the Department of Health agency linked to drugs and alcohol?
9   Name two types of psychological intervention used for drug and alcohol problems?
10 Name two differences in these types of intervention?

References

Alcohol Policy UK (2010) *Local alcohol profiles for England*, September issue. Available at http://www.alcoholpolicy.net/2010/09/local-alcohol-profiles-for-england-lape-2010-.html (accessed 26 June 2011).

Alcoholics Anonymous (2011) http://www.aa.org/lang/en/subpage.cfm?page=222 (accessed 24 June 2011).

Baker, M. and Buckley, D. (2011) Alcohol and mental health, in D.B. Cooper (ed.) *Practice in Mental Health – Substance Use*. London: Radcliffe.

Barker, P. and Buchanan-Barker, P. (2009) Getting personal: being human in mental health care, in P. Barker (ed.) *Psychiatric Nursing: The Craft of Caring*, 2nd edn. London: Hodder Arnold.

British Crime Survey (2009) Drug misuse declared: findings for the 2009/2010 British Crime Survey, in J. Hoare and D. Moon (eds) *Home Office Statistical Bulletin* (2010). Available at http://homeoffice.gov.uk/science-research/research-statistics/(accessed 15 June 2011).

British National Formulary (BNF) (2010) Available at www.bnf.org/bnf/extra/current/ 450003.htm#guideprescribing (accessed 7 June 2011).

Cooper, P.D. (2009) *The Person Who Experiences Mental Health and Substance Use Problems in Psychiatric Nursing: The Craft of Caring*, 2nd edn, P. Barker (ed.). London: Hodder Arnold.

Department of Health (DH) (2004) Alcohol needs assessment research project. Available at http://www.dh.gov.uk/prod_consum_dh/groups/dh_digitalassets/@dh/@en/documents/ digitalasset/dh_4122239.pdf (accessed 28 June 2011).

Department of Health (DH) (2007) *Safe, Sensible and Social: The Next Steps in the National Alcohol Strategy*. London: DH.

European Monitoring Centre for Drugs and Drug Addiction (EMCDDA) (2009) *Annual Report*.

FRANK (2011) Independent government-funded website. Available at http://www. talktofrank.com/drugs (accessed 20 June 2011).

Frischer, M., Crome, I., MacLeod, J. Bloor, R. and Hickman, S. (2005) *Predictive Factors for Illicit Drug Use Among Young People: A Literature Review*. London: Home Office. Available at http://www.ncjrs.gov/App/Publications/abstract.aspx?ID=240320 (accessed 20 June 2011).

HM Government (2008) *Drugs: Protecting Families and Communities – the 2008 Drug Strategy*. London: Central Office of Information.

Kipping, G. (2004) The person who misuses drugs or alcohol, in I. Norman and I. Ryrie (eds) *The Art and Science of Mental Health Nursing: A Textbook of Principles and Practice*. Maidenhead: Open University Press.

Kumpfer, K.L. and Bluth, B. (2004) Parent/child transactional processes predictive of resilience of vulnerability to 'substance abuse disorders', *Substance Use and Misuse*, 39: 671–98.

Marsden, J., Strang, J., Lavoie, D., Abdulrahim, D., Hickman, M. and Scott, S. (2004) Drug misuse, in A. Stevens, J. Rafferty, J. Mant and S. Simpson (eds) *Health Care Needs Assessment: The Epidemiologically Based Needs Assessment Reviews*. Oxford: Radcliffe.

McLoughlin, D. and Long, A. (1996) An extended literature review of health professionals' perceptions of illicit drugs and their clients who use them, *Journal of Psychiatric and Mental Health Nursing*, 3(5): 283–8.

Miller, S. and Rollnick, W.R. (2002) *Motivational Interviewing: Preparing People for Change*. New York: Guilford Press.

National Institute for Health and Clinical Excellence (NICE) (2007) *Drug Misuse Psychosocial Interventions – NICE Clinical Guideline 51*. London: National Institute for Health and Clinical Excellence.

National Institute for Health and Clinical Excellence (NICE) (2011) *Alcohol-use Disorders, Diagnosis, Assessment and Management of Harmful Drinking and Alcohol Dependence – NICE Clinical Guideline 115*. London: National Institute for Health and Clinical Excellence.

National Treatment Agency (NTA) (2006) *Models of Care for Adult Drug Misusers Updated*. London: NTA Publications.

National Treatment Agency (NTA) (2007) *Models of Care for Alcohol Misusers*. London: NTA Publications.

Prescott, C.A., Madden, P.A.F. and Stallings, M.C. (2006) Challenges in genetic studies of the etiology of substance use and substance use disorders: introduction to the special issue, *Behavior Genetics*, 36: 473–82.

Prochaska, J.O. and Diclemente, C.C. (1986) Toward a comprehensive model of change, in W.R. Miller and N. Heather (eds) (1998) *Treating Addictive Behaviours: Processes of Change*. New York: Plenum Press.

Rassool, G.H. (1998) Contemporary issues in addiction nursing, in G.H. Rassool (ed.) (2011) *Understanding Addiction Behaviours: Theoretical & Clinical Practice in Health and Social Care*, Basingstoke: Palgrave Macmillan.

Rassool, G.H. (2006) Nursing students perception of substance use and misuse, *Nursing Times*, 102(44): 33–4.

Rassool, G.H. (2007) Some considerations on attitude to addictions: waiting for the tide to change, *Journal of Addictions Nursing*, 18(2): 61–3.

Rassool, G.H. (2011) *Understanding Addiction Behaviours: Theoretical & Clinical Practice in Health and Social Care*. Basingstoke: Palgrave Macmillan.

Sellick, S. and Redding, B.A. (1998) Knowledge and attitudes of registered nurses towards perinatal substance abuse, *Journal of Obstetric, Gynaecologic & Neonatal Nursing*, 27(1): 70–7.

Treasure, J. (2004) Motivational interviewing, *Advances in Psychiatric Treatment*, 10: 331–7.

United Nations Office on Drugs and Crime (UNODC) (2009) *World Drug Report 2007*. Available at http://www.unodc.org/documents/about-unodc/AR06_fullreport.pdf (accessed 26th June 2011).

Wilson, I. (2011) Helping people who misuse substances, in S. Pryjmachuk (ed.) *Mental Health Nursing: An Evidences Based Introduction*. London: Sage.

World Health Organization (WHO) (1994) *International Classification of Diseases – 10*. Available at http://www.who.int/classifications/icd/en/ (accessed 20 June 2011).

7 Psychological interventions in learning disability and mental health

Karen Rea and James Ridley

Chapter aim and objectives

Aim

- To explore psychological interventions within a learning disability and mental health context.

Objectives

- To introduce the key issues that occur when learning disability is contextualized within the mental health field.
- To describe and critique the evidence base underpinning the care of individuals with a learning disability and mental health needs.
- To describe, analyse and apply psychological interventions to the care of individuals with a learning disability and mental health needs.

An introduction to learning disability and mental health

Having a learning disability does not confer immunity from having a mental health problem; according to Hatton (2002), 25 per cent to 40 per cent of the population of people with a learning disability experience a mental health problem. The accurate identification of prevalence rates for mental illness in people with learning disabilities is difficult due to the fact that there are no universally agreed prevalence statistics (Ballinger et al., 1991; Raghavan et al., 2004; Raghavan and Patel, 2005; Smiley, 2005). However, even with great differences within the prevalence data it remains acknowledged that the learning disabled population are more likely to suffer from psychiatric problems than the general population, and on this basis there is a need for the appropriate skills and services to be in place (Borthwick-Duffy, 1994; Matson and Sevin, 1994; DoH, 2006a; 2006b; NMC, 2010).

Having a learning disability is a lifelong condition. In 2001 it was estimated that there were approximately 1.5 million people within the UK diagnosed with a learning disability; this represented almost 2 per cent of the entire population (Foundation for People with Learning Disabilities, 2001). It is widely recognized that people with learning disabilities have much greater health needs than the general population, and alongside this is the recognition that this population also suffers from a greater range of health inequalities, such as access to services (Michaels, 2008).

Historically, people with learning disabilities have been perceived as requiring support from just learning disability specific services. Certainly for many years services such as long-stay institutions helped perpetuate this view as people rarely left the hospital grounds for any form of treatment or primary care. However, this viewpoint has moved on significantly with the publishing of documents such as the *National Service Framework for Mental Health* (DoH, 2001a), *Clinical Guidelines 1* (NICE, 2002) and *Valuing People* (DoH, 2001b), all of which clearly identify that access to health services should be equal, including mental health services. To support mental health services the Foundation for People with Learning Disabilities (2001) developed a range of guidance as well as an audit tool to help services establish how accessible they were to people with learning disabilities; this document is known as the 'Green-light tool kit' (DoH, 2004).

When supporting a person with a learning disability it is important to be able to recognize what this label means and how it can affect the individual, especially when planning care and/or attempting therapeutic interventions. There are many different interpretations and definitions related to learning disability, some of which are used for medical or psychological purposes. These definitions currently are to be found within classification resources such as *The ICD-10 Classification of Mental and Behavioural Disorders* (WHO, 1992) and the *Diagnostic and Statistical Manual of Mental Disorders* (DSM IV) (APA, 1994), both of which continue to be used. The term 'learning disability' was adopted following an agreement to move away from the label 'mental handicap' (DoH, 1992).

The most commonly used definition of learning disability can be found within the *Valuing People* white paper: 'A significantly reduced ability to understand new or complex information, to learn new skills (impaired intelligence). A reduced ability to cope independently (impaired social functioning), which started before adulthood, with a long lasting effect on development' (DoH, 2001b: 6).

Once it is identified that a person has a learning disability it is likely that some reference will be made to the severity or degree of their disability. A person is likely to be identified as having a mild, moderate, severe or profound learning disability (Hardy et al., 2006). The use of these sub-classifications does move away from the fact that the individual and their associated needs need to be person centred and holistic, however these terms are still commonly used (RCN, 2007). In relation to the care and treatment of individuals within these groups, there are likely to be quite significant differences in relation to the planning of an assessment, proposed treatment and other related interventions for mental illness.

A term used within mental health services and learning disability services which can cause confusion is 'dual diagnosis'. Within learning disability services this can be used to refer to a person who has a learning disability and a mental health problem; this can also refer to a person who presents with complex behaviour or who has another diagnosis, such as epilepsy. Therefore, where this term may be identified within case notes or patient documents, it will require further scrutiny at the initial assessment stage. This is of particular importance as within Mental Health Services the term 'dual diagnosis' most commonly refers to mental health problems complicated by substance misuse (see Chapter 6).

Some of the issues that need to be considered when completing any form of assessment with an individual who has a learning disability and a mental health problem are listed below.

- Individual's attention span/distractibility.
- Acquiescence – individuals agreeing based on the notion that this is what you want them to say. This can also be attributed to a person's level of understanding, basing their answers on the non-verbal cues given by the assessor rather than the question itself.
- Support staff as informants – these staff may have limited knowledge of mental health problems in general or how this can impact on the individual with learning disabilities.
- Carers change frequently – leading to a lack of detailed knowledge of changes in functioning.
- The individual may already have underlying cognitive deficits and impaired living skills, therefore functional decline may be difficult to identify.
- Prone to increased health problems, which may mimic psychiatric symptoms.
- Lack of communication skills to report on symptoms experienced.
- Rational for the assessment – is it the person, those around them, or could it be a re ion to the person's environment?

The following scenario overview provides a sense of what these issues may look like within the practice setting; the issues particular to the scenario will be explored further in the psychological interventions section.

SCENARIO

Thomas is a man with a moderate learning disability; he is 60 years of age. Thomas has been referred to the local Community Learning Disability Team (CLD). The referrer has stated that the reason for the referral is because of an increase in Thomas's agitated behaviour towards his support staff and his fellow tenants, and his very low mood. Thomas has been known to the community team in the past and has been seen by psychiatry on a number of occasions, but it was agreed after a previous admission to an acute mental health ward that the staff in the residential unit would in future make the initial referral to the local CLD services.

Alongside recognizing the importance of the issues identified above is the increasing awareness of the value and necessity of using evidence-based assessment tools, which will be explored in greater detail in the next section (Raghavan et al., 2004; Devine and Taggart, 2008).

Evidence-based practice

A key stage in working with individuals who have a learning disability and mental health needs is the assessment stage (DoH, 2006a). When completing an assessment it is important to ensure that you have covered the main areas in order to effectively use that information to plan care. A structured assessment framework or holistic assessment should enable the assessor to gain a variety of information, some of which may not have been given by a staff team or individual without a formal request. In agreement with Deb et al. (2001) the following would be some of the baseline information required to progress to an intervention, however this approach is not 'set in stone' and could be extended to include other assessments or measures, which ensures that a comprehensive assessment is then completed:

- family history
- personal history
- developmental history
- medical history
- psychiatric history
- social history
- drug history
- forensic history
- history of presenting complaint.

One critical issue related to the completion of any assessment and the subsequent intervention is the need to address the person's capacity and their ability to offer informed consent. In situations where a person's capacity is under question, it is likely that this assessment will require a truly person-centred approach. The Mental Capacity Act (2005) emphasizes the need to make every effort to support the person in making a decision. It *must* be remembered that a person who has a learning disability has exactly the same rights under the Mental Capacity Act (2005) and the Human Rights Act (1998) as any other citizen, and does not lose those rights for being informed in relation to all aspects of their care. Alongside this is the fact that the giving of this information may lead to the individual refusing the care offered.

The types of support required to ensure that people have the opportunity to make an informed decision may take the form of verbal and non-verbal techniques, including simplified language, line drawings, photographs and sign language (Evers, 2008). A clinician working with a person who has a learning disability is likely to need to adapt their communication skills accordingly; possibly even needing to outsource services and resources that ensure the information reflects what the individual may need in respect to giving informed consent. It is important to remember that individuals may not be able to fully articulate their information needs, and therefore patients and health professionals may have different perceptions of the important issues (Bowles, 1996). However, the benefits of clear information are significant; a person who is well informed is more likely to manage their situation/treatment, have better psychological outcomes and experience fewer exacerbations of their condition (Caress, 2003).

In relation to known risk factors for those who develop mental health problems, people with learning disabilities again are not immune. Factors such as unemployment, abuse, poverty, drug and alcohol problems, and discrimination are becoming more recognized as impacting factors on this population (DoH, 2009). Alongside this is an increased recognition that where a person has an additional impairment then the risk of developing mental health problems also increases (Gilbert et al., 1998). A study by Gilbert et al. (1998) identified that when someone has an additional impairment such as hearing, visual impairments or epilepsy, there is an increased risk of developing mental health problems. As has been found with other health-related needs, the learning disabled population has a higher prevalence of sensory impairments (Carvill, 2001), which needs to be considered in relation to a person's vulnerability to the development of mental health problems.

Just like the general population, people with learning disabilities can suffer from the full range of mental health problems (Hardy and Bouras, 2002), however certain characteristics related to a person's specific learning disability can predispose them to an increased risk of developing certain mental health conditions.

> *Schizophrenia:* according to O'Hara and Sperlinger (1997) the prevalence of schizophrenia, or what may be referred to as a 'psychotic disorder', is three times more likely in the learning disabled population.
>
> *Mood disorders:* it is estimated that the prevalence of mood disorders in people with learning disabilities is between 1.3 per cent and 3.7 per cent (Hardy and Bouras, 2002).
>
> *Anxiety disorders:* there are no estimates given for the amount of people given this diagnosis; however it is believed that, in line with other areas of research, the incidence of this within the learning disabled population is higher than the general population (Stavrakaki, 1999).
>
> *Dementia:* the prevalence rates for people with dementia are clearly showing that people with a learning disability are at a greater risk than the general population based on age (Cooper, 1997). Specific research related to people with Down's syndrome has found that they have a greater likelihood for developing what is termed 'early onset dementia', this typically relates to Alzheimer's disease. People with Down's syndrome are also found to show a higher prevalence of depression (Hardy and Bouras, 2002).

Chapters 3, 4 and 9 provide more information regarding these mental health problems. If we recognize that individuals with a learning disability often experience mental health problems it is important to identify how services respond to this need.

According to Devine and Taggart (2008) the most traditional approach to the care and treatment of a person with a learning disability who has a mental health problem is to use medication or behavioural approaches. The chosen approach is usually defined by the 'diagnosis' or group of symptoms; a behavioural approach is chosen when the information given to the staff team appears to suggest that the symptoms have a behavioural component. The term 'challenging behaviour' is commonly cited by services to explain a range of issues which they are finding difficult. The use of this label can significantly delay or mislead an assessment situation which may otherwise lead to a potential diagnosis of a mental illness. The term is defined as: 'Culturally abnormal behaviour(s) of such an intensity, frequency or duration that the physical safety of the person or others is likely to be placed in serious jeopardy, or behaviour which is likely to seriously limit use of, or result in the person being denied access to, ordinary community facilities' (Emerson, 1995: 20).

However, the need to ensure that the interventions used encompass a 'multi-modal' or holistic approach is vital for the care of this client group; using behavioural approaches may be a part of an intervention plan but should not be the sole focus of the individual's plan. In fact, the plan should encompass changes in the person's environment, improved communication and social skills training, as well as the use of appropriate medications (Taggart and Slevin, 2006). As previously discussed, there are a number of factors that can be attributed to the development of mental health problems in a person with learning disabilities; therefore, the need to use a variety of approaches will be required to support the individual (DoH, 2006a; 2006b). Devine and Taggart (2008) identify that no specific intervention was likely to produce long-term positive outcomes, so the need for those involved in the intervention planning to use a full range of approaches becomes absolutely vital.

When working with clients who have learning disabilities and mental health problems it is necessary to be cognizant of the issues that impact on the person's ability to engage in therapy. These include:

- referral and consent
- accessibility of therapy
- assessment
- confidentiality
- the therapeutic relationship
- communication
- interventions.

Once the client and/or carer has negotiated their way through the above issues, according to a report produced in 2004 by the Royal College of Psychiatrists, the commonly offered treatment to people with learning disabilities was that of cognitive behavioural therapy (CBT). Other therapeutic modalities were identified as being offered and these included:

- counselling and family counselling
- bereavement work
- supportive therapy
- specific work with Asperger syndrome
- psychodynamic psychotherapy
- brief, solution focused
- psychosexual

- vocational guidance
- art and music
- anger management and social skills
- play therapy
- working through carers
- integrative
- gestalt
- dialectical behaviour therapy
- psycho-educational work
- systemic
- transactional analysis
- sexual abuse counselling
- working with sex offenders (adapted from the Royal College of Psychiatrists, 2004).

Cognitive behavioural therapy was selected to help Thomas address his identified problems and the next section of the chapter will explore this in more depth.

Psychological interventions and scenario

Thomas is a client of a community learning disability team; he has had several admissions into acute mental health services and so is well known to both service providers. His admissions to a local acute mental health service in the past have been due to severe depression and/or challenging behaviour. The intention of this section is to provide information into possible reasons for Thomas's depression and to provide evidence of how Thomas can be helped to manage and resolve his problems.

Certainly some of these issues were apparent in relation to working with Thomas. Initial attempts at completing the assessment were met with him showing signs of increased anxiety, low-level verbal aggression and a total reluctance to engage; this included Thomas refusing to speak about his moods as well as any other issue. As a result there was a significant need for reliance on information gained from the staff team. This is often a common need and method for gaining information relating to an individual with a learning disability (Matousova-Done and Gates, 2006; Evers, 2008).

An area of the therapeutic work undertaken with Thomas which caused great difficulty was asking Thomas to engage in physical health screening; this was required so that it could be established whether he was suffering from any underlying physical condition or discomfort that may have been impacting on his mood. This took a significant amount of time to undertake as Thomas was reluctant to access local GP services. This was an important element of the baseline assessment process as one of the concerns was that Thomas at times was suffering from urinary incontinence. Owing to this, the team made attempts to engage Thomas in giving a urine sample which could rule out possible infection, as well as blood tests to rule out prostate difficulties and diabetes. The importance of identifying any physical health problems is not a new concept both for people with learning disabilities and people with mental health problems. It is identified that these groups are more likely to experience 'diagnostic overshadowing', that is reports of physical ill health being viewed as part of the mental health problem or learning disability and so not investigated or treated (Disability Rights Commission, 2006). However in relation to Thomas it was also essential to identify that his behaviour and mood were not being affected by an unknown physical health issue which may have required further support or simple treatment.

When an individual is presenting with challenging behaviour, it is likely that the assessment process for mental health problems becomes more difficult (Emerson et al., 1999), as was the case for Thomas. Research related to the presentation of challenging behaviour and its links to mental health problems has suggested that behaviours can be masking an undiagnosed psychiatric disorder (Smiley, 2005). However, Thomas would also use his behaviours to avoid or escape engaging with others. Therefore, a holistic approach towards Thomas's mental health became equally important, as Thomas's behaviours were having a significant negative impact on his quality of life.

Protective factors such as good relationships and activities can help a person who may have mental health problems (Grant et al., 2008). However if a person's behaviours mean that they lose out on these then the potential for a 'vicious circle' of challenging behaviour and mental distress could begin (Westbrook et al., 2007; Grant 2010). Certainly this was an issue that needed to be considered with Thomas. His behaviours were impacting on his relationships with his support staff and the men he was sharing with. What needed to be clarified was whether these behaviours were as a result of his low mood or as a reaction to other stimuli such as his environment, support or other issues as mentioned previously. The potential for a confused diagnosis and therefore intervention does raise the point of 'diagnostic overshadowing'. Within the context of challenging behaviour this term may be referred to as 'behavioural overshadowing' where the behaviours are simply attributed to the person's learning disability (Woodward and Halls, 2003) and not assessed appropriately for their function or cause.

A number of approaches were required to support Thomas. These included the completion of an assessment and planned interventions for his physical health and mental health as well as his behaviour (Smiley, 2005). As discussed previously the need for this holistic approach is required to ensure that the intervention plan enables all areas to be covered. Thomas's intervention plan showed a truly multidisciplinary approach: the professional links required to support Thomas included the use of nursing, psychiatry, speech and language therapy, occupational therapy and psychology. Based on the interventions of the groups, the staff were able to clearly identify their roles in the provision of an effective care package for Thomas.

The nurse involved worked as a care coordinator, but also led on the baseline assessments of Thomas's physical health, behaviour and mental health. The nurse completed a range of documents that related to mental health management (PRN protocol, relapse prevention plan), physical health (health needs assessment, health action plan, health passport) and behavioural support (proactive strategies, reactive strategies). These documents would be commonly used within the realms of a functional assessment, which is an assessment or a systematic investigation of the relationships between events in the environment and specific target behaviours (Paclawskyj et al., 2004).

As an example Thomas was asked about his view on his urinary incontinence, that is how did he feel about this, were there any problems with this health issue, what would he like to happen (Westbrook et al., 2007; Grant 2010)? The main problem as Thomas saw it was the ridicule he was subjected to by others regarding the smell and condition of his clothes. This made him feel very angry and ashamed. When he was asked what he would like to happen Thomas replied 'not to smell any more, and for people to leave me alone'. The staff worked with Thomas to identify why the problem was happening; this took the form of a diary, which Thomas and his care coordinator worked on producing together. The diary produced clear evidence as to why Thomas was occasionally incontinent, which then led to strategies being devised to manage this and to Thomas being reassured that there was no further need for medical interventions.

The completion of this diary over a week identified a clear pattern. Thomas was only incontinent of urine following a large fluid intake; he often did not respond to physiological sensations, that is the urge to void his bladder, especially if he was comfortable, and these factors led to urinary incontinence. The staff worked with Thomas on identifying the pros and cons of continuing in this way – a technique often used in problem solving (Grant, 2010) – and a behavioural plan was agreed.

1   Thomas would reduce his fluid intake before going to bed. This immediately led to a cessation in nocturnal enuresis.
2   Following the success of this behaviour change, Thomas agreed to 'listen' to his body's signals d go to the toilet as soon as he felt the urge to urinate. An additional posi. 'e outcome of this was a reduction in name calling, with a corresponding reduction in his aggressive behaviour. Thomas has since asked for help regarding personal hygiene and social skill development in washing his clothes.

Looking at Thomas's past it was also identified that, at times when his mood appeared to be low or he was displaying some form of agitation, he would refer to missing his parents. The team were able to identify, with the support of the psychologist, that this meant more than just his parents, but the family as a unit. Again the use of CBT proved very useful to clearly identify what the problems were for Thomas and how these could be addressed. The psychologist was able to give staff an insight into the grieving process for Thomas, but was also able to work directly with Thomas. This led to Thomas being able to discuss his feelings in relation to this, and the staff supporting him to build albums and collages of family pictures was also a benefit.

Using a vicious cycle approach enabled Thomas and the staff team to both manage the situation and also to look for collaborative ways to reduce Thomas's level of distress. This meant that alongside all of the interventions related to medication, staff training, and so on, the team always identified Thomas's role both with the planning process and the delivery of any associated interventions.

To ensure that this approach was truly collaborative it was important to identify Thomas's level of comprehension. By doing this the team were not only making sure that any information presented to Thomas was specific to his needs, but also that the communication process was thoughtful and person centred. The impact of being sensitive to Thomas's communication needs was that the interventions supported by the staff team were less likely to cause any significant confusion or distress and therefore less likely to exacerbate Thomas's mental health problems or behaviours.

Summary of the key points

It is important to acknowledge that the learning disabled population are more likely to suffer from mental health problems than the general population.

Mental health nurses need to be aware that using the term dual diagnosis can cause confusion if not clarified.

There are a number of therapies that can be offered in the treatment of people with learning disabilities and mental health needs; the most commonly used approach is cognitive behavioural therapy.

Using the vicious cycle approach allows the mental health nurse to work with people with learning disabilities and mental health needs to both collaboratively manage care and reduce distress.

Quick quiz

1   What range of percentages has been identified as the number of people with learning disabilities who have a mental health problem?
2   What is the name of the toolkit identified by the Foundation for People with Learning Disabilities?
3   What are the classifications of learning disability?
4   What does the term 'dual diagnosis' refer to in the context of learning disability and mental health problems?
5   What information is required when undertaking a mental health assessment of an individual with a learning disability?
6   What support/techniques are suggested by Evers (2008) in order to ensure that that the individual with a learning disability has the opportunity to make an informed decision?
7   What is the traditional approach to the care and treatment of a person with a learning disability who also has a mental health problem?
8   What issues may have an impact on a person's ability to engage in therapy?
9   What is the most commonly used therapeutic treatment for people who have a learning disability, according to the Royal College of Psychiatrists?
10   What is a functional assessment?

References

American Psychiatric Association (APA) (1994) *Diagnostic and Statistical Manual of Mental Disorders*, 4th edn. Washington, DC: APA.

Ballinger, B.R., Ballinger, C.B., Reid, A.H. and McQueen, E. (1991) The psychiatric symptoms, diagnoses and care needs of 100 mentally handicapped patients, *British Journal of Psychiatry*, 158: 255–9.

Borthwick-Duffy, S.A. (1994) Epidemiology and prevalence of psychopathology in people with mental retardation, *Journal of Consulting and Clinical Psychology*, 62(1): 17–27.

Bowles, L. (1996) How much should patients be told about their medication? *British Journal of Nursing*, (5)3: 157–64.

Caress, A.L. (2003) Giving information to patients, *Nursing Standard*, 17(43): 47–54.

Carvill, S. (2001) Sensory impairments, intellectual disability and psychiatry, *Journal of Intellectual Disability Research*, 45(6): 467–83.

Cooper, S.A. (1997) Epidemiology of psychiatric disorders in elderly compared with younger adults with learning disabilities, *British Journal of Psychiatry*, 170: 375–80.

Deb, S., Mathews, T., Holt, G. and, Bouras, N. (2001) *Practice Guidelines for the Assessment and Diagnosis of Mental Health Problems in Adults with Intellectual Disability*. Brighton: Pavilion.

Department of Health (DoH) (1992) *Health Services for People with Learning Disabilities (Mental Handicap) – HSG (92)42*. Leeds: NHS Executive.

Department of Health (DoH) (2001a) *National Service Framework for Mental Health*. London: DoH.

Department of Health (DoH) (2001b) *Valuing People: A New Strategy for Learning Disability in the 21st Century*. London: DoH.

Department of Health (DoH) (2004) *Valuing People Support Team, National Institute for Mental Health: Green Light for Mental Health; a Service Improvement Tool Kit*. London: DoH.

Department of Health (DoH) (2006a) *From Values to Action: The Chief Nursing Officer's Review of Mental Health Nursing*. London: DoH.

Department of Health (DoH) (2006b) *Best Practice Competencies and Capabilities for Pre-registration Mental Health Nurses in England: The Chief Nursing Officer's Review of Mental Health Nursing*. London: DoH.

Department of Health (DoH) (2009) *Valuing People Now: A New Three Year Strategy for People with Learning Disabilities*. London: DoH.

Devine, M. and Taggart, L. (2008) Addressing the mental health needs of people with learning disabilities, *Nursing Standard*, 22(45): 40–8.

Disability Rights Commission (2006) *Equal Treatment: Closing the Gap*. Stratford-upon-Avon: DRC.

Emerson, E. (1995) *Challenging Behaviour: Analysis and Intervention in People with Learning Disabilities*. Cambridge: Cambridge University Press.

Emerson, E., Moss, S. and Kiernan, G. (1999) The relationship between challenging behaviour and psychiatric disorders in people with severe developmental disabilities, in N. Bouras (ed.) *Psychiatric and Behavioural Disorders in Developmental Disabilities and Mental Retardation*. Cambridge: Cambridge University Press.

Evers, C. (2008) Assessing capacity: developing an integrated care pathway, *Learning Disability Practice*, 11(1): 30–3.

Foundation for People with Learning Disabilities (FPLD) (2001) *Learning Disabilities: The Fundamental Facts*. London: FPLD.

Gilbert, T., Todd, M. and Jackson, N. (1998) People with learning disabilities who also have mental health problems: practice issues and directions for learning disability nursing, *Journal of Advanced Nursing*, 27: 1151–7.

Grant, A. (ed.) (2010) *Cognitive Behavioural Interventions for Mental Health Practitioners*. Exeter: Learning Matters.

Grant, A., Townend, M., Mills, J. and Cockx, A. (2008) *Assessment and Case Formulation in Cognitive Behavioural Therapy*. London: Sage Publications.

Hardy, S. and Bouras, N. (2002) The presentation and assessment of mental health problems in people with learning disabilities, *Leaning Disability Practice*, 5(3): 33–8.

Hardy, S., Woodward, P., Woolard, P. and Tait, T. (2006) *Meeting the Health Needs of People with Learning Disabilities: Guidance for Nursing Staff*. London: RCN.

Hatton, C. (2002) Psychosocial interventions for adults with intellectual disabilities, and mental health problems, *Journal of Mental Health*, 11(4): 357–73.

Human Rights Act (1998) www.legislation.gov.uk/uk/ukpga/1998/42/contents.

Matousova-Done, Z. and Gates, B. (2006) The nature of care planning and delivery in intellectual disability nursing, in B. Gates (ed.) *Care Planning and Delivery in Intellectual Disability Nursing*. Oxford: Blackwell.

Matson, J.L. and Sevin, J.A. (1994) Theories of dual diagnosis in mental retardation, *Journal of Consulting and Clinical Psychology*, 62(1): 6–16.

Mental Capacity Act (2005) www.dca.gov.uk/legal-policy/mental-capacity/mca-summary.pdf.

Michaels, J. (2008) *Healthcare for All: Report of the Independent Inquiry into Access for Healthcare for People with Learning Disabilities*. London: Aldridge Press.

National Institute for Clinical Excellence (NICE) (2002) *Clinical Guidelines 1: Schizophrenia – Core Interventions in the Treatment and Management of Schizophrenia in Primary and Secondary Care*. London: NICE.

Nursing and Midwifery Council (NMC) (2010) *Standards for Pre-registration Nursing Education*. London: NMC.

O'Hara, J. and Sperlinger, A. (1997) Mental health needs, in J. O'Hara and A. Sperlinger (eds) *Adults with Learning Disabilities: A Practical Approach for Health Professionals*. Chichester: John Wiley and Sons.

Paclawskyj, T.R., Kurtz, P.F. and O'Connor, J.T. (2004), Functional assessment of problem behaviours in adults with mental retardation, *Behaviour Modification*, 28: 649–67.

Raghavan, R. and Patel, P. (2005) *Learning Disabilities and Mental Health: A Nursing Perspective*. Oxford: Blackwell.

Raghavan, R., Marshall, M., Lockwood, A. and Duggan, L. (2004) Assessing the needs of people with learning disabilities and mental illness: development of the learning disability version of the Cardinal Needs Schedule (LDCNS), *Journal of Intellectual Disability Research*, 48(1): 25–36.

Royal College of Nursing (RCN) (2007) *Mental Health Nursing of Adults with Learning Disabilities*. London: Royal College of Nursing.

Royal College of Psychiatrists (2004) *Psychotherapy and Learning Disability: Council Report*. London: Royal College of Psychiatrists.

Smiley, E. (2005) Epidemiology of mental health problems in adults with a learning disability: an update, *Advances in Psychiatric Treatment*, 11(3): 214–22.

Stavrakaki, C. (1999) Depression, anxiety and adjustment disorders in people with intellectual disabilities, in N. Bouras (ed.) *Psychiatric and Behavioural Disorders in Developmental Disabilities and Mental Retardation*. Cambridge: Cambridge University Press.

Taggart, L. and Slevin, E. (2006) Care planning in mental health settings, in B. Gates (ed.) *Care Planning and Delivery in Intellectual Disability Nursing*. Oxford: Blackwell.

Westbrook, D., Kennerly, H. and Kirk, J. (2007) *An Introduction to Cognitive Behavioural Therapy: Skills and Applications*. London: Sage Publications.

Woodward, P. and Halls, S. (2003) Staff training in the mental health needs of people with learning disabilities in the UK, *Advances in Mental Health and Learning Disabilities*, 3(2): 15–19.

World Health Organization (1992) *The ICD-10 Classification of Mental and Behavioral Disorders: Clinical Descriptions and Diagnostic Guidelines*. Geneva: WHO.

8 Psychological interventions and working with families

Paula Kennedy

Chapter aim and objectives

Aim
- To explore the context and application of family therapy approaches to working with families of those experiencing mental health problems.

Objectives
- To identify systemic family therapy applications as they apply in mental health care practice.
- To describe and critique the evidence base underpinning family therapy interventions.
- To describe, analyse and apply family therapy to a scenario related to a young person and his family.

An introduction to working with families

As mental health nurses, we must 'Work with others to protect and promote the health and wellbeing of those in your care, their families and carers, and the wider community' (NMC, 2008: 5).

The first part of this chapter will explore the context of working with families in mental health practice using a family therapy approach. The second part of the chapter will look at the evidence base for family therapy, and the third part of the chapter will explore the application of family therapy within a scenario. 'Building and maintaining positive interpersonal relationships with service users and carers is essential to successful mental health nursing practice. Specific interpersonal skills, the offering of meaningful choice and person-centred values all help build positive relationships (DH, 2006a: 26).

The importance of the inclusion of family members/carers in mental health care has been emphasized extensively in a plethora of standards and guidance available to the mental health practitioner (DH, 2002; 2006b; 2007a; 2007b; NMC, 2008; 2010; see also Figure 8.1). The focus of this has surrounded inclusion and the development

NICE (2011a) Anxiety: support families & carers
NICE (2011b) Alcohol Dependence & Harmful Alcohol use: brief strategic FT (BSFT); functional FT (FFT); multi-systemic FT (MST); multidimensional treatment for foster care (MTFC)
NICE (2011c) Common Mental Health Disorders: engage with & meet the needs of families and carers.
NICE (2010) Alcohol-Use Disorders: encourage families and carers to be involved in the treatment
NICE (2009c) Schizophrenia: family interventions; single family intervention; multi-family group interventions
NICE (2009a) Antisocial Personality Disorder: BSFT; FFT; MST; MTFC
NICE (2009b) Borderline Personality Disorder: involve families or carers
NICE (2008) ADHD: parental training programmes
NICE (2007) Drug Misuse: behavioural couples therapy; behavioural family interventions; social systems interventions
NICE (2006) Bi-polar Disorder: consider structured formal family interventions
NICE (2005b) OCD: offer family support for children with OCD
NICE (2005a) Depression in Children: shorter-term FT (systemic behavioural FT); systemic FT
NICE (2004) Eating Disorders: family interventions; eating disorder focused family therapy (FT); combined individual & family work

Figure 8.1 Family-inclusive standards and guidance

of therapeutic relationships to support both the service user and the people who are important in their lives.

Phases of 'experiences' that famil҆ ͐ go through in caring for members with mental health problems include: feeling overwhelmed (consumed); grief and loss; personal costs of caring; seeking knowledge and understanding; making sense of what is happening; and becoming empowered (Wynaden, 2007). Family members are often described as: 'Experiencing varying levels of powerlessness and invalidation in their interactions with mental health professionals' (Shanker and Muthesawamy, 2007: 306).

As expressed above, feelings of loss and grief are common in those caring for loved ones who are experiencing mental health problems, and are attributed to increased vulnerability to psychological and emotional distress for family members and carers (Dixon and Lehman, 1995; James et al., 2006; Lobban and Barrowclough, 2009; Maunu and Stein, 2010).

It may be of use at this juncture to identify the difference between the terms 'family therapy' and 'family interventions'. Family interventions offer service users and their families the opportunity to not only consider the impacts of their lived experience, but also ways in which they can support and be supported through what for many is a traumatic and life-changing experience. The term is commonly (but not exclusively) used when thinking about interventions for psychosis and schizophrenia (Lobban and Barrowclough, 2009). 'The elements of family interventions most frequently used in differing combinations are psycho-education, behavioural problem solving, family support, and crisis management' (Dixon and Lehman, 1995: 631).

In contrast, family therapy, while incorporating elements of the above definition, is a psychological intervention delivered by a qualified systemic family psychotherapist (AFT, 20011a; 2011b).

> Family and Systemic Psychotherapy – often called Family Therapy – helps people in close relationship help each other. It enables family members to express and explore difficult thoughts and emotions safely, to understand each other's experiences and views, appreciate each other's needs, build on family strengths and make useful changes in their relationships and their lives.
>
> (AFT, 2009a: 1)

Recovery is at the forefront of mental health care treatment and the relevance of families in the process of recovery is emphasized. 'The recovery paradigm in mental health acknowledges families as important players in the recovery process. Families are often at the centre of people's social worlds, providing them with primary support networks' (Piat et al., 2011: 50).

In summary, the purpose of this chapter is to explore complexity in relation to parental suicide for children and their carer's; the genogram (Figure 8.2) and scenario provide an illustrative example within mental health practice of the familial impact

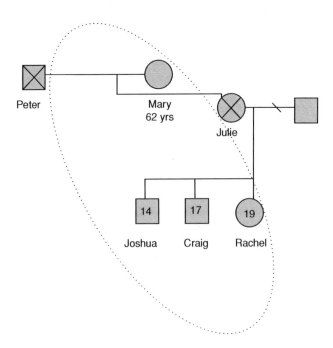

Figure 8.2 Scenario genogram

of adult mental health problems. We will look at this scenario in more detail in the psychological interventions section as they pertain to family therapy.

SCENARIO

Joshua is a 14-year-old young man who has been referred to the Child and Adolescent Mental Health (CAMH) psychological services following concerns raised by his GP and the school. Further to his Child and Mental Health Service (CAMHS) assessment Joshua was diagnosed as suffering from 'socialized conduct disorder' and a request was made for individual and family therapy interventions.

Joshua lives with his maternal grandmother following the death of his mother through suicide when he was 11 years old. Joshua has two older siblings: a brother (Craig) aged 17 years and a sister (Rachel) aged 19 years, all of whom live with their maternal grandmother. The children have no contact with their biological father, who left when Julie was pregnant with Joshua. Joshua has been described in the referral has having difficulties in managing his behaviour and emotions, being verbally aggressive, disobedient, running away from home frequently, misusing alcohol and illicit substances (cannabis mainly) and acting without consideration of the consequences.

His school experience is also affected as he misses lessons and feels that his concentration is poor. The relationships between family members are often fraught with tension and outbursts of aggression. Mary has described feeling that she is no longer able to 'cope' with Joshua.

Evidence-based practice

In thinking about Joshua and his family it would be helpful to first identify the components and evidence base for systemic family therapy, followed by the evidence base as it applies to his individual diagnosis of conduct disorder and the family's context in terms of bereavement as a result of suicide and kinship care. All of these aspects will be explored in greater detail as we move through the section.

Systemic family therapy

Some of the principles that underpin systemic family therapy practice have been included to provide a context for the evidence base specific to Joshua's family scenario. 'A systemic approach postulates that if family dynamics change, individual identity and experience can change alongside it and vice versa; if an individual changes, his or her relationships will also change' (Garvin and White, 2009: 198). The family is often structured by its relationship to itself, which may also be shaped by current or historic multigenerational influences and its environment which includes intrinsic values and expectations that may exist (Garvin and White, 2009; Nichols, 2010).

Families move through transitional phases or 'lifestyle cycles', much like the people within them. The ability to adjust to these changes can create contextual challenges for some families (Carr, 2006; Dallos and Draper, 2010).

> Presenting difficulties are not seen as fixed or residing within an individual but as framed by the surrounding network of relationships and beliefs. This allows us to be less pathologising of individuals as we become more aware of the effects of patterns and how they can hold individuals in place. A contextual view, offering a wider field of vision can therefore trigger more ideas for both the therapist and the family.
>
> (Garvin and White, 2009: 202)

Through conversation, the family and the therapist are able to view situations from multiple perspectives creating a context for change; the creation of multiple perspectives is facilitated in the exploration of relationships and meaning, using such techniques as conversational partnerships and circular questioning (among others). We will explore these techniques in the next section of the chapter as they apply to Joshua and his family (Gergen, 1994; Madsen, 1999; Anderson, 2001; 2005; Vetere and Dallos, 2003; Nichols, 2011).

During the 1980s and 1990s Harlene Anderson, Harry Goolishian, Lynn Hoffman and others developed ideas that moved from biological constructivist ideology to social constructionist ideology (Flaskas, 1997). 'The power of social interactions is in generating meaning for people...our beliefs are fluid and fluctuating in relation to context...no one has the corner on truth, all truths are social constructions' (Nichols, 2011: 215). In this context the role of therapy was one of exploration of the derivation of the families' world view, language and interaction make possible the families' ability to create new constructions and therefore possibilities. To be collaborative means that no 'one truth' is presented. Rather dialogue enables the emergence of shared new realities (Gergen 1991; Nichols, 2011).

Systemic family therapy has developed over the past decade and a growing evidence base has emerged as to its efficacy. As we have seen, this is implicit in many of the National Institute for Clinical Excellence (NICE) guidelines for practice (2004; 2005a; 2005b; 2006; 2007; 2008; 2009a; 2009b; 2009c; 2010; 2011a; 2011b; 2011c). Current implications for practice focus on its inclusion within further guidelines for evidenced-based practice (Stratton, 2005; Carr, 2010).

Conduct disorder and systemic family therapy

To set the context for intervention as it relates to systemic family therapy, Joshua's diagnosis of conduct disorder (CD) should be explored. Conduct disorder is seen as a disorder of development of behaviour. Factors that lead to this are many and complex. The ICD-10 (WHO, 1992) suggest six sub-groups; one of the groups is socialized CD, which is the diagnosis given to Joshua. Children diagnosed with socialized CD are generally well integrated in their peer group; it is the relationships they have with adults (particularly those in authority) that tend to be poor. Behaviour related to a diagnosis of CD may first appear at school and coincide with deterioration in the quality of the child's school work. Where it first appears during adolescence, behaviours manifest within the wider community and criminal activities may develop (WHO, 1992).

The ICD-10 lists 15 behaviours in the diagnosis of CD. An individual needs to have had at least three of these behaviours manifest during the past 12 months for diagnosis to take place. Joshua is described as having the following behaviours:

- bullying, threatening or intimidating others (usually his siblings or people in his social circle)
- initiating physical fights (again this is towards his siblings and outside of the home within the local community)
- deliberately destroying others' property by other means (he has a police caution for damage to a motor vehicle, his grandmother's)
- theft of items of non-trivial value without confrontation of a victim (has stolen from his grandmother)
- staying out late at night frequently, despite parental prohibition, beginning before age 13
- running away from home overnight at least twice, or once without returning for a lengthy period
- often truanting from school, before age 13 (WHO, 1992).

Factors that impact upon the development of CD are varied and complex, however research has suggested that: 'Paternal psychopathology and the quality of the relationship between mother and child may pose risk specifically for comorbid CD' (Pfiffner et al., 2005: 551).

The National Institute for Health and Clinical Excellence is in the process of developing guidelines specific to CD. The outcome in terms of evidence-based treatments is yet to be established, however 'Multisystemic therapy is a well-established, empirically supported treatment for adolescent conduct disorder or juvenile delinquency' (Carr, 2010: 410).

Suicide-bereaved families and systemic family therapy

'Suicide should be seen not as a sudden isolated disaster but as a major event in an unhappy series, bringing in its wake grief certainly, but the possibility also of relief' (Shepherd and Barraclough, 1976: 272). Joshua's family are living with the aftermath of parental suicide, limited literature specific to this and its impact upon the family was identified, however literature specific to suicide or bereavement and children enables a collation of themes: 'The Child course of bereavement can be particularly sensitive to a number of complicating factors: developmental tasks, the surviving parent's warmth and care-giving ability, the influence of stigma, and family environment, including the manner of communication surrounding the death' (Hung and Rabin, 2005: 782).

Responses to loss and bereavement in children and young people include, post-traumatic stress disorder, depression, guilt and self-blame, and high-risk behaviours. Joshua presents with high-risk behaviours:

> Suicide-bereaved children were more likely to have pre-existing behavioural problems and more behavioural and anxiety symptoms in the first 2 years after the death compared with those bereaved by other causes. They were also more likely to experience anger at 6 months, shame at 1 year, and less acceptance between 1 and 2 years after the death than those bereaved by other causes.
>
> (Hung and Rabin, 2009: 785)

The role of shame experienced in combination with stigma can result in limiting social support (Breen and O'Connor, 2011). Pre-existing vulnerabilities indicate risks for the family in their response to loss through suicide, challenging the family's entire belief system, including their own sense of themselves as a unit. Families bereaved by suicide are less liable to talking about their loss, however sharing their experiences provides a space in which others may feel more able to talk (Wertheimer, 2001).

> The effects of loss on the family system will depend on the role the deceased played within the family and whether the death leaves a gap which someone else must now fill. The emotional integration of the family will affect the degree to which its members can help one another cope, and whether families value or hinder communication, particularly when it comes to expressing emotions.
>
> (Worden, 1991, in Wertheimer, 2001: 95)

Kinship care and systemic family therapy

Joshua and his siblings have been cared for by their maternal grandmother; this family care arrangement is also known as 'kinship care'. In 2008, 71 per cent of 'looked after children' in the UK were in foster care placements. Of that number, 11 per cent were cared for by family (ONS, 2009). Much of the literature surrounding kinship care originates from the USA, however it is broadly defined as: 'The full-time nurturing and protection of children who must be separated from their parents, by relatives, members of their tribes or clans, godparents, stepparents, or other adults who have a kinship bond with a child' (CWLA, 1994: 2).

Kinship care is said to 'enable children to live with persons whom they know and trust, it reduces the trauma children may experience when they are placed with persons who are initially unknown to them, and reinforces children's sense of identity and self esteem which flows from their family history and culture' (Wilson and Chipungu, 1996: 387).

The 'rock and the hard place' when referring to kinship care is often a term used by families, particularly those in positions of caring for children (Ziminski, 2006; 2007a; 2007b; Sandfield and Gopfert, 2010). Themes and dilemmas from the literature that may be considered in relation to Joshua and his family may include the following.

1 *Themes*
   - Complex legal systems.
   - Fragility of kinship carers' mental and physical health: in what way has Mary's mental/physical health been affected following the death of her daughter and her subsequent care of three children?
   - Outcomes of 'kinship care' are generally better than those for foster care.
2 *Dilemmas*
   - Feelings of guilt about how they may have supported the parent and child 'better'.
   - Complex family dynamics/roles: unresolved trauma, understanding inter-generational family dynamics.
   - Extended family: resource or source of conflict?
   - Conflicting parenting values between mum Julie and grandmother Mary.

Psychological interventions and scenario

In relation to the chapter scenario, this section will look at systemic family therapy interventions all of which take into account the evidence base as described in the evidence base section of this chapter. We will explore the use of systemic formulation and alliance building alongside collaborative therapy and post-Milan techniques.

Systemic formulation

'The formulation we develop about a family can be thought of as a story we have created to organize our thinking in order to be helpful to that family. Our formulation is not "objective truth" but one of a number of possible stories' (Madsen, 2007: 81). For Joshua and his family the formulation could include the following statement:

> Following the loss of their mother/daughter who suffered with a chronic de-pressive illness and subsequently completed suicide, multiple factors have contributed to the family's difficulties in relating to and communicating with one another about their loss. Fear surrounding stigma and blame may hold them back from having such conversations. The complexity that surrounds formal kinship care arrangement has compounded their struggles, and sub-sequent feelings of hopelessness and despair about the future have emerged. Joshua's response to the traumatic experiences of loss have served as a means of enabling the family to consider their relationships and ways of communicating through therapy.

You may wish to revisit and reformulate this as the exploration of the families context unfolds during the remainder of this section.

Therapeutic alliance

'To really understand the history of the family and the family as it now exists, family therapists have to talk with the whole family . . . children can offer the therapist a good indication of the emotional climate of the family' (Rober, 2008: 465). Engaging Joshua and his siblings in the initial and subsequent sessions would be a key component in the process of alliance building not only with them as family members but also as young adults. Young people need to feel that the therapeutic space is safe enough for them to talk, particularly when talking about issues that may not have been spoken about (Lever and Gmeiner, 2000). Acknowledging and exploring with family members their understanding of family therapy and how they came to be at the session may enable Joshua and his siblings to establish a voice. Children can be apprehensive about coming to therapy, worried or anxious; they may have tensions about wanting to be heard but feeling safe to talk, wanting to be respected for their views and 'feeling comfortable' (Moore and Bruna Seu, 2011).

One of the early questions the therapist may ask of themselves is in what ways can I make the session safe for Joshua, Craig and Rachel, but also grandmother, Mary? Understanding further the impact of loss through exploration of the evidence base may be a resource in contextualizing the complexity of grief through suicide, one which may be compounded by many unanswered questions, feelings of helplessness and responsibility combined with feelings of anger and blame.

'Another way in which families become engaged from the beginning of the therapeutic process is by careful introduction of the family and all the therapists involved, as well as a full and understandable explanation of the roles of the different participants and the way of working in that particular context' (Lever and Gmeiner, 2000: 46). Introductions during initial sessions enable the therapist to draw on the client's strengths and resources as well as establish what challenges the family face; the therapist would hope to take a collaborative stance in developing the therapeutic alliance with Joshua and his family, and would aim to identify some sense of a shared understanding about goals. One of the mechanisms for asking exploratory introductory questions is in the use of circular questions.

A collaborative approach

A collaborative approach is recommended when working with families in 'out of home' placements such as kinship care or foster placement (Sparks and Muro, 2009), this would form the basis of a rationale for identifying a collaborative systemic family therapy approach to working with Joshua and his family.

Collaborative approaches constitute a philosophy, stance or way of being providing an umbrella under which several theoretical models may sit (Madsen, 1999; Anderson, 2001; Fraenkel, 2006). The definition of a therapeutic stance makes the identification of collaborative skills tricky and while techniques (by virtue intervention) are not described in the literature it does depict some contextual components, described as a set of 'characteristics' that become guidelines for practice:

- Conversational partnerships
- Clients as experts
- Not knowing
- Being public
- Mutual transformation
- Uncertainty
- Everyday ordinary life (Anderson, 2005).

In relation to Joshua and his family, the component of conversational partnership will be explored.

Conversational partners take equal responsibility in dialogue; the therapist and clients invite this approach to take place. Tentative therapeutic questions taken directly from the dialogue are part of this partnership approach, with the aim being to expand upon or say the unsaid (Anderson and Goolishian, 1992; Anderson, 2001). An example of this might be: during a discussion between the therapist and Joshua, Craig suggests that Joshua 'takes' cannabis to be the 'big man in the house'. The therapist may then ask Joshua what he thinks Craig might mean by the term 'big man in the house', thus opening a space for family members to consider meaning and possibilities about how they understand the term, its origins (both familial and in the wider context) and its impact upon relationships, dialogue and behaviour. The question can be developed to ask for reflections from Craig on Joshua's understanding of meaning and also to explore others' perspectives. This technique of asking family members to comment on each other is known as circular questioning.

The technique of circular questioning originates from the work of the Milan team during the 1980s. Selvini et al. (1980) developed three principles of the Milan method: hypothesizing, neutrality and circularity. Central to these three principles was the technique of circular questioning (Brown, 2010). This shift saw the therapist as integral to the conversational system.

As we have already stated, the collaborative 'stance' acknowledges the expertise of the family. However, the family therapist also acknowledges that they are holding and presenting tentatively the things they might presuppose about the family (Anderson, 2005) which may be located within the therapist questions: 'A presupposition is what the question assumes. In most cases of natural conversations, the presuppositions carried in questions are not overtly stated, that is, they are embedded in the question' (McGee et al., 2005: 374).

In relation to issues of kinship care, the family therapist may become thoughtful about the 'dilemmas' (Ziminski, 2007a) that Joshua and his family may be experiencing, leading to a variety of presuppositions specific to the experiences of kinship carers:

- *Dilemma: choice and responsibility* Does Mary feel she has divided loyalties between her daughter's past and the children's search for answers? Between Joshua's need to develop his sense of his mother's story and Mary's need to protect Joshua and his siblings from this? Does this in any way connect with stories the family may have about mothers and motherhood? About death and loss?

- *Dilemma: loss and entitlement* Does Mary perceive herself as being blamed for Julie's loss? Do any other members of the family feel blame or blamed?
- *Dilemma: belonging and identity* How has Mary constructed the idea of family with Joshua, Craig and Rachel now, and what are her hopes for the future? What influences will sustain or negate those hopes?

Translating these presuppositions and wonderings into circular questions over time can assist in the exploration of the derivation of Joshua's families world view to make possible the family's ability to create new constructions and therefore possibilities (Nichols, 2011).

From the position of a collaborative stance, the therapist would aim to ensure that questions came from the story and language used by the family. For example, in relation to ideas about loss, Rachel wondered about a question Joshua had asked her a few years ago about him being the reason for mum dying. The therapist may presuppose that Joshua's question was a means of checking out one or even all of the dilemmas above.

In response to Rachel's wonderings, the therapist may ask a circular question, such as 'Rachel, when Joshua asked you about being the reason for his mother dying what do you think may have led him to this conclusion?' In asking this question I am inviting Rachel to draw on some connections (Brown, 1997) in terms of meaning between herself and Joshua about the ideas surrounding responsibility and loss.

Tentative therapeutic questions taken directly from the dialogue would enable a more collaborative approach, the therapist's aim being to expand upon or expose the unsaid (Anderson and Goolishian, 1992; Anderson, 2001). Circular questions are inherently therapeutically more effective than lineal questions (Tomm, 1988). 'In contrast to linear questions circular questions obtain information about differences between people, events, relationships or beliefs' (Loos and Bell, 1990: 47). Circular questions generate and liberate, enabling the therapist and family to move away from reductionist perceptions supported by lineal questioning and on to a more collaborative exploration of the family's story from multiple perspectives (Tomm, 1988; Dozier et al., 1998; Ingham, 2011).

Summary of the key points

Systemic principles acknowledge the cyclical nature of communication and relationships. As mental health nurses the influence of linear models of thinking about the challenges that the people we work with face can restrict our ability to create opportunities that may exist for families to change and develop.

Family therapy has a growing and recognized evidence base in the interventions for families whose members may have been identified as experiencing mental health problems across a range of contexts and settings.

Developing an appreciative collaborative stance with families enables the development of therapeutically effective relationships, resulting in positive outcomes.

Some of the techniques and skills used in systemic family therapy practice are accessible and transferable to the mental health nurses in everyday practice; however, the integration of systemic family therapists in child and adult mental health practice has proved an effective resource in the delivery and consultation processes involved in psychological interventions.

Quick quiz

1   What are the 'phases' a family may go through in caring for a member with mental health problems?
2   How might you define the role of the family therapist?
3   Name the NICE guidelines where family therapy is the recommended choice of treatment?
4   What is a systemic formulation NOT?
5   What factors might a family therapist consider in engaging young people in family therapy?
6   What are the seven characteristics of the collaborative approach?
7   What are the benefits of circular questions in contrast to linear questions?
8   What type of circular question might you ask of Mary regarding the 'big man of the house'?
9   What would you hope the outcomes of developing a collaborative stance with families might be?
10 Can you develop the original formulation and identify what presuppositions may be driving this?

References

Anderson, H. (2001) Postmodern collaborative and person centred therapies: what would Carl Rogers say? *Journal of Family Therapy*, 23(4): 339–60.

Anderson, H. (2005) A postmodern collaborative approach to therapy: broadening the possibilities of clients and therapists. Available at http://www.harleneanderson.org/writings/postmoderncollaborativeapproach.htm.

Anderson, H. and Goolishian, H. (1992) The client is the expert: a not-knowing approach to therapy, in S. McNamee and K.J. Gergen (eds) *Therapy as Social Construction*. London: Sage Publications.

Association for Family Therapy and Systemic Practice in the UK (AFT) (2009) *Building Family Strengths: What is Family Therapy?* Warrington: AFT. Available at http://www.aft.org.uk/home/documents/Leafletindd.pdf.

Association for Family Therapy and Systemic Practice in the UK (AFT) (2011a) *Code of Ethics and Practice*. Warrington, AFT.

Association for Family Therapy and Systemic Practice in the UK (AFT) (2011b) *Summary of Family Interventions Recommended and Reviewed in NICE Guidelines: Update*. Warrington: AFT.

Breen, L.J. and O'Connor, M. (2011) Family and social networks after bereavement: experiences of support, change and isolation, *Journal of Family Therapy*, 33: 98–120.

Brown, J. (1997) Circular questioning: an introductory guide, *Australian and New Zealand Journal of Family Therapy*, 18(2): 109–14.

Brown, J.M. (2010) The Milan principles of hypothesising, circularity and neutrality in dialogical family therapy: extinction, evolution...Or emergence? *Australia and New Zealand Journal of Family Therapy*, 31(3): 248–65.

Carr, A. (2006) *Family Therapy: Concepts, Process and Practice*, 2nd edn. Chichester: Wiley.

Carr, A. (2010) Thematic review of family therapy journals, *Journal of Family Therapy*, 32(4): 409–27.

Child Welfare League of America (CWLA) (1994) *Kinship Care: A Natural Bridge*. Washington, DC: Child Welfare League of America.

Dallos, R. and Draper, R. (2010) *An Introduction to Family Therapy; Systemic Theory and Practice*, 3rd edn. Maidenhead: Open University Press.

Department of Health (2002) *Developing Services for Carers and Families of People with Mental Illness*. London: Department of Health.

Department of Health (2006a) *From Values to Action: The Chief Nursing Officer's Review of Mental Health Nursing*. London: Department of Health.

Department of Health (2006b) *Best Practice Competencies and Capabilities for Pre-registration Mental Health Nurses in England: The Chief Nursing Officer's Review of Mental Health Nursing*. London: Department of Health.

Department of Health (2007a) *Best Practice in Managing Risk: Principles and Guidance for Best Practice in the Assessment and Management of Risk to Self and Others in Mental Health Services*. London: Department of Health.

Department of Health (2007b) *Independence, Choice and Risk: A Guide to Best Practice in Supported Decision Making*. London: Department of Health.

Dixon, L.B. and Lehman, A.F. (1995) Family interventions for psychosis, *Schizophrenia Bulletin*, 21(4): 631–43.

Dozier, R.M., Hicks, M.W., Cornille, T.A. and Peterson, G.W. (1998) The effect of Tomm's therapeutic questioning styles on therapeutic alliance: a clinical analog study, *Family Process*, 37: 189–200.

Flaskas, C. (1997) Reclaiming the idea of truth: some thoughts on theory in response to practice. *Journal of Family Therapy*, 19(1): 1–20.

Fraenkel, P. (2006) Engaging families as experts: collaborative family program development, *Family Process*, 45(2): 237–57.

Garvin, R. and White, H. (2009) Key systemic ideas as seen through the eyes of first-year trainees, *Australian and New Zealand Journal of Family Therapy*, 30(3): 196–215.

Gergen, K. (1991) The saturated family, *Family Therapy Networker*, 15: 26–35.

Gergen, K. (1994) *Realities and Relationships: Soundings in Social Construction*. Cambridge, MA: Harvard University Press.

Hung, N.C. and Rabin, L.A. (2009) Comprehending childhood bereavement by parental suicide: a critical review of research on outcomes, grief processes, and interventions, *Death Studies*, 33(9): 781–814.

Ingham, B. (2011) Collaborative psychosocial case formulation development workshops: a case study with direct care staff, *Advances in Mental Health and Intellectual Disabilities*, 5(2): 9–15.

James, C., Cushway, D. and Fadden, G. (2006) What works in engagement of families in behavioural family therapy? A positive model from the therapist perspective, *Journal of Mental Health*, 15(3): 355–68.

Lever, H. and Gmeiner, A. (2000) Families leaving therapy after one or two sessions: a multiple descriptive case study, *Contemporary Family Therapy*, 22(1): 39–65.

Lobban, F. and Barrowclough, C. (eds) (2009) *A Casebook of Family Interventions for Psychosis*. Chichester: Wiley-Blackwell.

Loos, F. and Bell, J.M. (1990) Circular questioning: a family interviewing strategy, *Dimensions of Critical Care Nursing*, 9(1): 47–53.

Madsen, W.C. (1999) *Collaborative Therapy with Multi-stressed Families*. New York: Guilford Press.

Madsen, W.C. (2007) *Collaborative Therapy with Multi-stressed Families*, 2nd edn. New York: Guildford Press.

Maunu, A. and Stein, C.H. (2010) Loss of having a parent with mental illness: young adults' narrative accounts of spiritual struggle and strength, *Journal of Community Psychology*, 38(5): 645–55.

McGee, D., Del Vento, A. and Beavin-Bavelas, J. (2005) An intentional model of questions as therapeutic interventions, *Journal of Marital and Family Therapy*, 31(4): 371–84.

Moore, L. and Bruna Seu, I. (2011) Giving children a voice: children's positioning in family therapy, *Journal of Family Therapy*, 33(3): 279–301.

National Institute for Clinical Excellence (NICE) (2004) *Eating Disorders: Core Interventions in the Treatment and Management of Anorexia Nervosa, Bulimia Nervosa and Related Eating Disorders – Clinical Guideline 9*. London: National Institute for Clinical Excellence.

National Institute for Clinical Excellence (NICE) (2005a) *Depression in Children and Young People: Identification and Management in Primary, Community and Secondary Care – Clinical Guideline 28*. London: National Institute for Clinical Excellence.

National Institute for Clinical Excellence (NICE) (2005b) *Obsessive-compulsive Disorder: Core Interventions in the Treatment of Obsessive-compulsive Disorder and Body Dysmorphic Disorder – Clinical Guideline 31*. London: National Institute for Clinical Excellence.

National Institute for Health and Clinical Excellence (NICE) (2006) *Bipolar Disorder: The Management of Bipolar Disorder in Adults, Children and Adolescents, in Primary and Secondary Care – Clinical Guideline 38*. London: National Institute for Health and Clinical Excellence.

National Institute for Health and Clinical Excellence (NICE) (2007) *Drug Misuse: Psychosocial Interventions – Clinical Guideline 51*. London: National Institute for Health and Clinical Excellence.

National Institute for Health and Clinical Excellence (NICE) (2008) *Attention Deficit Hyperactivity Disorder: Diagnosis and Management of ADHD in Children, Young People and Adults – Clinical Guideline 72*. London: National Institute for Health and Clinical Excellence.

National Institute for Health and Clinical Excellence (NICE) (2009a) *Antisocial Personality Disorder Treatment, Management and Prevention – Clinical Guideline 77*. London: National Institute for Health and Clinical Excellence.

National Institute for Health and Clinical Excellence (NICE) (2009b) *Borderline Personality Disorder: Treatment and Management – Clinical Guideline 78*. London: National Institute for Health and Clinical Excellence.

National Institute for Health and Clinical Excellence (NICE) (2009c) *Schizophrenia: Core Interventions in the Treatment and Management of Schizophrenia in Adults in Primary and Secondary Care (Update of NICE Clinical Guideline 1) – Clinical Guideline 82*. London: National Institute for Health and Clinical Excellence.

National Institute for Health and Clinical Excellence (NICE) (2010) *Alcohol-use Disorders: Diagnosis and Clinical Management of Alcohol-related Physical Complications – Clinical Guideline 100*. London: National Institute for Health and Clinical Excellence.

National Institute for Health and Clinical Excellence (NICE) (2011a) *Generalised Anxiety Disorder and Panic Disorder (With or Without Agoraphobia) in Adults: Management in Primary, Secondary and Community Care (Updates and Replaces NICE Clinical Guideline 22) – Clinical Guideline 113*. London: National Institute for Health and Clinical Excellence.

National Institute for Health and Clinical Excellence (NICE) (2011b) *Alcohol-use Disorders: Diagnosis, Assessment and Management of Harmful Drinking and Alcohol Dependence – Clinical Guideline 115*. London: National Institute for Health and Clinical Excellence.

National Institute for Health and Clinical Excellence (NICE) (2011c) *Common Mental Health Disorders: Identification and Pathways to Care – Clinical Guideline 123*. London: National Institute for Health and Clinical Excellence.

Nichols, M.P. (2010) *Family Therapy: Concepts and Methods*, 9th edn. Boston, MA: Pearson Education.

Nichols, M.P. (2011) *The Essentials of Family Therapy*, 5th edn. Boston, MA: Pearson Education.

Nursing and Midwifery Council (2008) *The Code: Standards of Conduct, Performance and Ethics for Nurses and Midwives*. London: Nursing and Midwifery Council.

Nursing and Midwifery Council (2010) *Standards for Pre-registration Nursing Education*. London: Nursing and Midwifery Council.

Office for National Statistics (ONS) (2009) *Social Trends: 39*. Available at http://www.statistics.gov.uk/downloads/theme_social/Social_Trends39/Social_Trends_39.pdf (accessed 10 April 2011).

Pfiffner, L.J., McBurnett, K., Rathouz, P.J. and Judice, S. (2005) Family correlates of oppositional and conduct disorders in children with attention deficit/hyperactivity disorder, *Journal of Abnormal Child Psychology*, 33(5): 551–63.

Piat, M., Sabetti, J., Fleury, M.-J., Boyer, R. and Lesage, A. (2011) Who believes most in me and in my recovery: the importance of families for persons with serious mental illness living in structured community housing, *Journal of Social Work in Disability and Rehabilitation*, 10(1): 49–65.

Rober, P. (2008) Being there, experiencing and creating space for dialogue: about working with children in family therapy, *Journal of Family Therapy*, 30: 465–77.

Sandfield, G. and Gopfert, M. (2010) Grandparents looking after grandchildren: between a rock and a hard place, *Context*, 108: 20–3.

Selvini Palazzoli, M., Boscolo, L., Cecchin, G. and Prata, G. (1980) Hypothesizing, circularity, neutrality: three guidelines for the conductor of the session, *Family Process*, 19(1): 3–12.

Shankar, J. and Muthuswamy, S.S. (2007) Support needs of family caregivers of people who experience mental illness and the role of mental health services, *Families in Society*, 88(2): 302–10.

Shepherd, D.M. and Barraclough, B.M. (1976) The aftermath of parental suicide for children, *British Journal of Psychiatry*, 129: 267–76.

Sparks, J.A. and Muro, M.L. (2009) Client directed wraparound the client as a connector in community collaboration, *Journal of Systemic Therapies*, 28(3): 68–76.

Stratton, P. (2005) *Report on the Evidence Base of Systemic Family Therapy*. Warrington: Association for Family Therapy.

Tomm, K. (1988) Interventive interviewing: part 111: intending to ask lineal, circular, strategic, or reflexive questions? *Family Process*, 27: 1–15.

Vetere, A. and Dallos, R. (2003) *Working Systemically with Families: Formulation, Intervention and Evaluation*. London: Karnac.

Wertheimer, A. (2001) *A Special Scar: The Experiences of People Bereaved by Suicide*, 2nd edn. Hove: Brunner-Routledge.

Wilson, D.B. and Chipungu, S.S. (1996) Introduction special edition: kinship care, *Child Welfare*, 75(5): 387–95.

Worden, J.W. (1991) *Grief Counseling and Grief Therapy*, 2nd edn. New York: Springer.

World Health Organization (WHO) (1992) *The ICD-10 Classification of Mental and Behavioral Disorders*. Geneva: WHO.

Wynaden, D. (2007) The experience of caring for a person with a mental illness: a grounded theory study, *International Journal of Mental Health Nursing*, 16: 381–9.

Ziminski, J. (2006) Who has the last word? Professional and family authority in the kinship care of children, *Context*, 87: 53–4.

Ziminski, J. (2007a) Dilemmas in kinship care: negotiating entitlements in therapy. *Journal of Family Therapy*, 29: 438–53.

Ziminski, J. (2007b) Systemic practice with kinship care families, *Journal of Social Work Practice*, 21(2): 239–50.

9 Psychological interventions and working with the older adult

Denise Parker

Chapter aim and objectives

Aim

- To explore the biopsychosocial issues of working with older adults experiencing mental health problems, including proposed causes and interventions.

Objectives

- To identify older people's mental health, particularly dementia, in terms of theories, approaches and classification.
- To describe and critique the evidence base underpinning the care of individuals with dementia.
- To describe, analyse and apply psychological interventions to the care of individuals with dementia.

An introduction to working with the older adult

The first part of this chapter will explore older people's mental health, focusing particularly on dementia. One of the challenges for staff working both within and outside the National Health Service (NHS) is the need to respond to the needs of the ageing population. Traditionally, older adults have been defined as being aged 65 and over (Eliopoulos, 2010). However, the origin of age 65 signalling old age is cloaked in controversy. Historically, since the late nineteenth century, it has been to do with the pensionable age (Roebuck, 1979). As people are living longer, this inevitably means that the incidences of people experiencing conditions such as dementia have also increased (DoH, 2009). Working with older people with mental health conditions and their carers is often challenging, particularly when symptoms take the form of behaviour that is difficult to cope with, such as in dementia. Evidence-based strategies for working with older people and their carers require an understanding of their individual experience and to enhance the quality of life of the older person. This chapter engenders a process of development through promoting the opportunity for you to focus on developing your skills and knowledge in working in this area of care, and by further encouraging you to value and respect the privacy, dignity and cultural diversity of the individual, encountered as part of your working lives.

The care of the older adult speciality has been blighted by workers often being paid low salaries, and a lack of research activity (Kitwood, 1997). Older people with mental health problems are more likely than younger people to have multiple diagnoses of physical health problems (DoH, 2001a). Psychological interventions for use with people with mental health conditions are already covered elsewhere in this book; these interventions are the same for older people with mental health problems. However, it is important for the practitioner to consider the person as an individual, and not to lose sight of the fact that older people have a lifetime of coping with life events. The context and psychosocial interventions needed for each person needs to be given attention, for example the 'baby boomers' (the post-war generation born between the late 1940s until 1963) are now coming into the 'older adult' age group. They have only ever known the welfare state and the NHS. Their expectations and lifestyle may be different from people born a generation earlier. 'Older people' are not a homogenous group. They are more likely than younger people to have been bereaved of a close relative or partner, or to have debilitating physical illness. Other issues may be the ageing process itself – we are a society that values youth. For example, an older person may have based their self-worth in a youthful self-image. When this is compromised, the person's self-esteem may take a blow. Older people may experience loss on several levels: youth, close ones (either literally or through geographical distance), work, perceptions of usefulness and lifestyle. Evidence suggests that cognitive behavioural therapy (CBT) is successful for the treatment of many mental health conditions (DoH, 2001b). The same report recommends that:

a) The patient's age, sex social class or ethnic group are generally not important factors in choice of therapy and should not determine access to therapies.

b) Ethnic and cultural identity should be respected by referral to culturally-sensitive therapists.

(DoH, 2001b: 35)

The National Service Framework for Older People (DoH, 2001a) Standard Seven is about mental health in older people, but interestingly it really concentrates only on depression and dementia. This infers that older people do not experience the full range of mental health problems experienced by younger people. However, it is important to be mindful of the impact of the 'three Ds' on older people's mental health – depression, dementia and delirium.

There are many types of organic disorder. In fact, the majority of people experiencing organic disorders are treated outside of specialist mental health services. It is therefore important to have an overview of signs, symptoms and treatments. The major feature of organic disorders is one of impaired cognitive functioning. There are many causes for delirium, including infection (urine or chest commonly), high temperature, side effects of medication, withdrawal suddenly from drugs or alcohol, liver or kidney dysfunction, brain injury, terminal illness and constipation (RCP, 2009). Delirium can be induced by psychoactive substances, such as alcohol. However, when these are not the cause:

A   There is clouding of consciousness, i.e. reduced clarity of awareness of the environment, with reduced ability to focus, sustain or shift attention.

B   Disturbance of cognition is manifest by both:
  1) impairment of immediate recall and recent memory,
  2) with relatively intact remote memory; disorientation of time, place and person.

C   At least one of the following psychomotor disturbances is present:
  1) rapid, unpredictable shifts from hypoactivity to hyperactivity:
  2) increased reaction time;
  3) increased or decreased flow of speech;
  4) enhanced startle reaction.

D   There is disturbance of the sleep or sleep–wake cycle, manifest by at least one of the following:
  1) insomnia, which in many cases may involve total sleep loss, with or without daytime drowsiness, or reversal of the sleep–wake cycle;
  2) nocturnal worsening of symptoms;
  3) disturbing dreams and nightmares, which may continue as hallucinations or illusions after awakening.

E   Symptoms have rapid onset and show fluctuations over the course of the day.

F   There is objective evidence from history, physical and neurological examination, or laboratory tests of an underlying cerebral or systemic disease (other than psychoactive substance-related) that can be presumed to be responsible for clinical manifestations in criteria A–D.

(World Health Organization, 1993a: 38–9)

Dementia is an umbrella term and is defined as:

A syndrome due to disease of the brain, usually of a chronic or progressive nature, in which there is disturbance of multiple higher cortical functions, including memory, thinking, orientation, comprehension, calculation, learning capacity and judgment. Consciousness is not clouded. The impairments of cognitive function are commonly accompanied, and occasionally preceded, by deterioration in emotional control, social behaviour or motivation. This syndrome occurs in Alzheimer's disease, in cerebrovascular disease, and other conditions primarily, or secondarily affecting the brain.

(World Health Organization, 1993b: 46)

The term dementia defines a group of syndromes characterised by progressive decline in cognition of sufficient severity to interfere with social and/or occupational functioning, caused by disease or trauma, and often associated with increasing age. To date, over 200 subtypes have been defined...

(Stephan and Brayne, 2008: 11)

Peters (2001) notes that there is considerable overlap in the pathology of types of dementia. This suggests that that mixed forms may be more common. The risk of dementia increases with age – up to 31 per cent of older people in hospital and 5 per cent of people living in the community are affected. People with Down's syndrome have a much higher risk of developing Alzheimer-type dementia – with an earlier onset age of 30–40 years. Approximately 55 per cent of people with Down's syndrome will be affected by dementia when aged 60–69 (compared with 5 per cent of the rest of the population). The prevalence of Alzheimer's and other forms of dementia in other people with learning disabilities is no greater than the rest of the population (DoH, 2005a): '821,884 people in the UK live with dementia. Dementia costs the UK economy £23 billion per year. This is more than cancer (£12 billion per year) and heart disease (£8 billion per year) combined' (Luengo-Fernandez et al., 2010: 11).

The National Institute for Clinical Excellence and the Social Care Institute for Excellence (NICE/SCIE, 2006) state that not everyone with memory problems has dementia; they may have mild cognitive impairment (MCI), which may not always progress to dementia. 'Primary healthcare staff should consider referring people ' to show signs of mild cognitive impairment (MCI) for assessment by memory assess. nt services to aid early identification of dementia, because more than 50% of people with MCI later develop dementia' (NICE/SCIE, 2006: 22).

To summarize this section, the following case scenario gives an example of how a diagnosis of dementia can have an impact on an individual and their significant others. This scenario will be revisited in more detail in the psychological interventions section.

SCENARIO

Jim is 72 years old and lives at home with his wife Joyce. They have grown-up children, Andrew and Pippa. Andrew lives 200 miles away. He has 4-year-old twins, Holly and Jade. They visit once a month. Pippa lives locally with her partner, Ant, and their son, Jack, aged 13. Jim is a retired gardener. Joyce is a part-time shop assistant. Since Jim retired, the couple have enjoyed many holidays in their caravan in Wales, and abroad. They particularly enjoy line dancing together and their social life at the golf club. The highlight of Jim's week is when Jack comes after school, and they go to the golf driving range. Jim says to Joyce often, as he cuddles up to her in bed, 'we didn't do

(continued)

too bad, did we girl? We got there in the end.' Joyce has heard this so many times before, but it is comforting to know that life has generally been good to them.

Jim's confusion exacerbated when he had a urinary tract infection. He was given antibiotics, and the confusion did lessen. However, when they visited Jim's GP, Joyce stated that 'things were not right' for a while. They informed the GP that, over the past few months, Jim's been a bit more irritable than usual, more frustrated. He agreed that he feels as if his mind is 'cotton wool' at times, and that he gets 'befuddled'. Joyce has noticed that he does not seem to be quite his perky self at times. Occasionally, his shirt buttons are fastened wrongly, and his concentration is not so good. He forgot to pick Jack up from school a couple of times, after promising him a lift. Jack was furious. Jim was embarrassed. He also is reluctant to go out, especially to line dancing, as he complains of having 'two left feet'. Joyce is frustrated too, as Jack seems to forget the steps of dances. She has accused him of being difficult deliberately. This causes rows. Then there was the incident the other day, when she asked Jim to put the lamb in the oven ready for when she came home. He did this, but had not bothered to switch the oven on. She shouted at him. Later she felt guilty, as she is beginning to realize that it is not always his fault.

Evidence-based practice

The evidence base for psychological interventions in dementia care is strengthening. Moniz-Cook and Manthorpe (2009) point out that there is a dearth of internationally accepted evidence-based psychological interventions for people with early dementia for practitioners to use. This, they indicate, is owing to problems of evidence-based practice in psychosocial intervention being difficult to achieve. They point out that where studies have been done, they tend to concentrate on the difficulties of caring for people with severe and disabling symptoms. 'Thus most dementia care intervention literature relates to family carer "burden", nursing home care or drug therapy' (Moniz-Cook and Manthorpe, 2009: 13).

Early diagnosis and intervention in dementia care is crucial (NICE/SCIE, 2006; DOH, 2009; Moniz-Cook and Manthorpe, 2009). However, this is at times hindered by a lack of knowledge about dementia (DOH 2009). It had been highlighted almost a decade earlier (Audit Commission, 2000) that only half of GPs thought it important to look actively for signs of dementia and make an early diagnosis. Also, there was a lack of clear information, and psychological support for both dementia sufferers and their carers (Audit Commission, 2000). Despite mounting evidence that things needed to improve, dementia care still has a long way to go. In 2009, the long anticipated report *Living Well With Dementia: A National Dementia Strategy* by the Department of Health came out, consolidating examples of good practice. It covers three key areas:

1   improved awareness
2   earlier diagnosis and interventions
3   a higher quality of care.

The strategy identifies 17 key objectives:

1   Improving public and professional awareness and understanding of dementia
2   Good quality diagnosis and intervention for all
3   Good quality information for people diagnosed with dementia and their carers
4   Enabling easy access to care, support and advice following diagnosis
5   Development of structured peer support and learning networks
6   Improved community personal support services
7   Implementing the Carers' Strategy
8   Improved quality of care for people with dementia in general hospitals
9   Improved intermediate care for people with dementia
10 Considering the potential for housing support, housing-related services and telecare to support people with dementia and their carers
11 Living well with dementia in care homes
12 Improved end-of-life care for people with dementia
13 An informed and effective workforce for people with dementia
14 A joint commissioning strategy for dementia
15 Improved assessment and regulation of health-care services and of how systems are working for people with dementia and their carers
16 A clear picture of research and evidence and needs
17 Effective national and regional support for implementation of the strategy

Much of the evidence base for psychological interventions in dementia care derives from person-centred care. Psychologist Tom Kitwood's writing on 'personhood' from the 1980s and 1990s remains influential in present-day dementia care. It has been suggested that had Kitwood survived to develop his theory, he would have adjusted some of his ideas, and acknowledged that his was a work in progress (Baldwin and Capstick, 2007). 'Personhood', as conceptualized by Kitwood, is a way to preserve the integrity, dignity and well-being of the person with dementia. He defined personhood as 'a standing or status that is bestowed on one human being by others, in the context of relationship and social being' (Kitwood, 1997: 5). Person-centred care, according to Kitwood, included valuing every human, regardless of age and cognitive impairment. Every person with dementia has a unique life story, life experience and response to dementia. They have their view of it, and relationships can contribute to their quality of life.

Personhood was discussed by Cantley (2001) as a term used to describe the essence of the whole person. Since the late 1980s person-centred care in dementia has valued the worth of each person regardless of age, illness or disability (Cantley, 2001). Kitwood developed the notion of Malignant Social Psychology based on his belief that the disease process of dementia disabled the person, but that what we do as a society disables them also. Kitwood (1997), NICE/SCIE (2006) and DOH (2009) stress the importance of carer support.

In the past 40 years, the main therapies used with people with dementia were reality orientation and reminiscence therapy. However, the evidence base for these therapies is weak. The evidence base for psychological interventions in dementia care is growing, particularly around cognitive stimulation therapy, and its contribution to slowing cognitive decline is comparable to drug therapy (NICE/SCIE, 2006). NICE/SCIE (2006) cites a credible evidence base for two types of therapy for the cognitive symptoms of Alzheimer's disease – one is pharmacological therapy via the use of the three acetylcholinesterase inhibitors: donepezil, galantamine and rivastigmine (but they are recommended only for people with moderate Alzheimer's disease). The other therapy is the psychological therapy, cognitive stimulation therapy. This is carried out in a group context and is an early intervention. 'Cognitive stimulation encompasses reality orientation, which focuses predominantly on current time and reminiscence therapy (RT) which focuses on past memories' (Oyebode and Clare, 2008: 159).

> People with mild-to-moderate dementia of all types should be given the opportunity to participate in a structured group cognitive stimulation programme. This should be commissioned and provided by a range of health and social care staff with appropriate training and supervision, and offered irrespective of any drug prescribed for the treatment of cognitive symptoms of dementia.
> (NICE/SCIE, 2006: 29)

Knapp et al. (2006: 579) concur that: 'CST groups have been shown to have beneficial effects on cognition and quality of life for people with dementia.' Spector et al. (2003) conducted a single-blind randomized controlled trial from multiple centres. The hypothesis was tested that CST for older adults with dementia would benefit cognition and quality of life. There were 115 people in the intervention group and 86 people in the control group. They concluded that their results compared favourably with trials for dementia drugs, and had benefits for many people with dementia.

Other psychological therapies apart from CBT in their own right do not have as strong an evidence base as CST. Cognitive training is another psychological intervention. It involves the person being given guidance to practise a set of tasks, reflecting particular cognitive functions, such as memory, attention and problem solving (Clare and Woods, 2003). Different methods can be used, such as paper and pencils, and computer programs, in varying settings (Clare and Woods, 2003; Oyebode and Clare, 2008). Cognitive training as carried out in studies has been intense, such as 30–60-minute sessions delivered three to seven times weekly by staff and carers (family) (Oyebode and Clare, 2008).

Cognitive rehabilitation is another psychological intervention, used on a one-to-one basis rather than group settings. It involves Kitwood's person-centred philosophy (Kitwood, 1997). Interventions are tailor-made, using knowledge of the person's cognition and behaviour. The aim is 'to improve quality of life and well-being through optimizing cognitive functioning in relation to everyday problems, and reduce excess disability' (Oyebode and Clare, 2008: 158). However, there is no evidence for the efficacy of cognitive training, and insufficient evidence for individualized cognitive rehabilitation, according to a systematic review by Clare and Woods (2003).

Other psychological therapies include working with life story. This is based on reminiscence therapy. This information enhances our chances of using person-centred interventions. Kitwood (1997) stressed that in order to understand a person with dementia, we need to know and understand their life history and their experience of dementia. We need to know their individual needs and behaviour. He indicated that dementia can cause ongoing trauma and distress, as the person has to contend with many losses (including identity) and changes. This is where life history work can be a useful tool in dementia care. However, the evidence base is weak. McKeown et al. (2005: 237) highlight that: 'It may help challenge ageist attitudes and assumptions, be used as a basis for individualized care, improve assessment, assist in transitions between different care environments, and help to develop improved relationships between care staff and family carers.' In their systematic review of the literature of life story work in health and social care, McKeown et al. (2005) concluded that there are research gaps, and there has been a lack of research into users' own experience of life-story work. The impact of it has been subjective depending on staff attitudes.

Psychological interventions and scenario

Jim's general practitioner had experience of working with people with dementia, as the practice staff had improved awareness of dementia in the last few years (Audit Commission, 2000; DoH, 2001a; 2009). He recognized that Jim's cognitive difficulties needed further assessment. He also recognized that Jim's difficulties with cognition could be due to mild cognitive impairment, but also dementia (WHO, 2003; NICE/SCIE, 2006). Following a couple of appointments at the surgery, where Jim had blood tests and a physical that ruled out delirium, infection and other physical causes for his cognitive deficits, he was referred to a memory clinic at the local hospital. DoH (2009) suggests that there should be better access to memory clinics. Fortunately, this is available in Jim's locality. A diagnosis was confirmed of Alzheimer's-type dementia (WHO, 2003). He scored 18 on the MMSE (Mini Mental State Examination) (Folstein et al., 1975). In keeping with NICE/SCIE (2006) guidelines, magnetic resonance imaging (MRI) was the preferred modality to help with early diagnosis, following consent by Jim. As he has mental capacity at present to consent to the diagnostic tests, the Mental Capacity Act (DoH, 2005b) is not required at this stage in Jim's dementia journey. However, as his condition progresses, eventually he would need more support. He may not be able later to make decisions for himself, and therefore the Mental Capacity Act (DoH, 2005b) must be used, and every effort made by his carers to enable him to make decisions for himself, and if in the event he cannot, then his best interests must be taken into account.

Following the diagnosis of Alzheimer's-type dementia, which came as devastating news to them, Jim and Joyce attended psychoeducational sessions arranged by the staff in the memory clinic on 'what is dementia' (Moniz-Cook and Manthorpe, 2009). These sessions clarified some practical issues, such as financial and support opportunities. Jim attended a cognitive stimulation therapy course; this consisted of 14 sessions, twice weekly over seven weeks, based on reminiscence therapy and reality orientation (Spector et al., 2003). These consisted of sessions on themes of physical games, sound, childhood, food, current affairs, faces/scenes, word association, being creative, categorizing objects, orientation, using money, number games, word games and a team quiz. Jim felt nervous at first meeting new people (Spector et al., 2003). However, the main benefit to Jim was the knowledge that he was not the only person experiencing difficulties similar to his, and this really helped him. For example, he felt so stupid when he fastened his shirt buttons up incorrectly on some days, but now he realizes that it happens to other people too. On such days, he may just need a bit more time and support. On other days, the shirt buttoning is not a problem.

Not long after diagnosis, Andrew, Jim's son, had come to visit. He told Jim and Joyce about support outside the statutory services. He mentioned the Alzheimer's Society. He has a colleague who gained a lot of support from her local Alzheimer's carer support group. On searching the Alzheimer's Society website, he found a lot of helpful information. This included leaflets on all kinds of things concerning possible support that people with dementia, and their families, needed, such as information leaflets, campaigns, events and research. Age UK, the Department of Health and Dementia UK websites were also very helpful. On the Dementia UK website, for example, he discovered that specialist dementia nurses existed, called Admiral Nurses. However, most useful were the information snippets on how to deal with challenges that the person with dementia and their family can face, such as 'wandering'. He also learnt that there are reasons behind different behaviours, and this has helped Andrew to understand his father. A diagnosis of dementia was devastating to Jim and his family, and he and Joyce were supported to come to terms with this by the multidisciplinary team, their family and support groups, such as one for carers run by the local branch of the Alzheimer's Society.

Jim was irritating Joyce by asking her 'constantly' what the date is. At home, cognitive training techniques were used (Clare and Woods, 2003; Oyebode and Clare, 2008). A calendar was put up on the wall with the date and day; each time that Jim enquired, Joyce pointed it out to him. She also used newspapers and a 24-hour clock. After a couple of weeks, Jim was asking less frequently and going straight to the calendar rather than asking Joyce the date. If he did ask, she would encourage him to find out for himself. However, Joyce realized that the calendar and newspapers must be in date, otherwise Jim would be further confused.

The GP and memory clinic staff, such as Katie, a community nurse who specialized in dementia care, encouraged Jim and Joyce to continue with their activities. Jim enjoyed his garden and, together, he and Joyce chose plants and drew up a list of things to do each week in the garden. By using this approach, the garden did not become too cumbersome for both Jim and Joyce. It was also something that they could do together. Seeing Jim taking pride in his garden gave Joyce so much pleasure. It also helped to raise Jim's self-esteem. As time went on, and Jim was less able to do so much in the garden, Joyce enlisted the help of a local gardener. However, she encouraged Jim to do as much as he was able to do.

Jim was given the opportunity to take anti-dementia medication for his Alzheimer's disease. His MMSE (Folstein et al., 1975) score was 15. He had been prescribed the acetylcholinesterase inhibitor donepezil (NICE/SCIE, 2006). Eventually, this pharmacological intervention stopped being as effective as his dementia worsened. It had, however, given Jim some respite from the disease. The benefit of him taking donepezil was that his cognitive functioning was maintained at a level whereby he was able to make decisions for himself, and experience a better quality of life with it than without it. When he had to stop taking it, Joyce and the family were very upset, as was Jim himself. Katie and the team explained the reasons why it had to be stopped, and although the family understood the rationale, it did not make it less upsetting for them.

As Jim's condition deteriorated, he needed to go into 24-hour care. It was important that the staff looking after him knew his likes, dislikes, strengths and areas where support was needed (Kitwood, 1997). He was not always settled in the residential home. He often wanted to go home, and would frequently ask 'Where is Joyce? I want to go home'. Cognitive rehabilitation (Oyebode and Clare, 2008) techniques were found to be quite helpful as Jim's dementia progressed. His family were asked to start a life-story book with Jim, and Joyce brought in some photographs and articles from home for his room. It was important that the staff in the care home had an understanding and knowledge of Jim's history, dementia experience and behaviour (Kitwood, 1997). A storyboard was put on his wall. An understanding of important relationships is crucial when caring for people with dementia. This informed interventions with Jim and his family (Nolan et al., 2004). An example of the importance of engaging with Jim, using knowledge from his life-story book and his family, was that if Jim was involved in gardening, his mood lifted, and he appeared to be more settled.

With the love, care and involvement of the family, and the care of professionals involved in his care, Jim was able to enjoy the best quality of life possible. Obviously, when Jim was coming towards the end of his life, this was a distressing time for his family, and the staff who had come to know him so well. However, good palliative care (DoH, 2009) meant that Jim had the best quality of life possible until the end of his life. A Macmillan nurse became involved in his care, and he had access to the cal hospice. The life-story book and story board helped to maintain the essence of who Jim is – his 'personhood' (Kitwood, 1997; Cantley, 2001; Nolan et al., 2004; Oyebode and Clare, 2008). The family were part of Jim's collaborative care, and remained involved in it until his passing. When he was no longer able to make decisions for himself, the decisions were made, in collaboration with the treatment team and his family, in Jim's best interests. This was because, as Jim's ability to make his own decisions deteriorated, along with his mental capacity, the Mental Capacity Act (2005) was used (DoH, 2005b). All throughout Jim's dementia journey, Joyce maintained contact with her local carer support group.

Summary of the key points

As mental health nurses, we are bound by a code of conduct to use non-discriminatory practice (NMC, 2008). Therefore, we must understand and put into practice the tenet that people cannot be discriminated against on the grounds of age (DoH, 2001a). People over the age of 65 have the same needs, aspirations, hopes, and right to dignity and privacy as younger people.

Dementia is an umbrella term. There are over 200 sub-types known so far. The most common types of dementia are Alzheimer's, vascular dementia and dementia with Lewy bodies. The most known types of fronto-temporal dementia include Korsakoff's psychosis, Pick's disease and Creutzfeldt–Jakob disease. The main risk of developing dementia is age.

Part of the problem with psychological interventions in dementia care is that often the evidence base is weak. However, the NICE/SCIE (2006) guidelines on dementia state that the two evidenced-based interventions with the strongest evidence are cognitive stimulation therapy and the pharmacological intervention of the use of acetylcholinesterase inhibitors, such as donepezil, galantamine and rivastigmine.

It is important to not forget that everything that we do as nurses is to maintain 'personhood' in the care of people experiencing dementia. We have to ensure that our patients have the best quality of life possible, and that we play an important part in making this achievable. This includes the consideration of good palliative care.

Quick quiz

1   Describe your understanding of dementia.
2   Identify the causes of delirium.
3   List the three main anti-dementia drugs used for people experiencing Alzheimer's-type dementia.
4   Compare and contrast the possible biopsychosocial differences between people of 65 years of age, and people of 85 years of age.
5   List the factors that could contribute to a person over 65 experiencing depression.
6   List the areas of support that a person newly diagnosed with dementia may need.
7   List the areas of support that the carer of a person with dementia living at home might need.

References

Audit Commission (2000) *Forget Me Not Report*. London, Audit Commission.
Baldwin, C. and Capstick, A. (2007) *Tom Kitwood on Dementia: A Reader and Critical Commentary*. Maidenhead: Open University Press.
Cantley, C. (2001) *A Handbook of Dementia Care*. Maidenhead: Open University Press.
Clare, L. and Woods, C. (2003) Cognitive rehabilitation and cognitive training for early-stage Alzheimer's disease and vascular dementia, *Cochrane Library, Cochrane Database of Systematic Reviews*, 4.
Department of Health (DoH) (2001a) *The National Service Framework for Older People*. London: Department of Health.
Department of Health (DoH) (2001b) *Treatment Choice in Psychological Therapies and Counselling. Evidence Based Clinical Practice Guideline*. London: Department of Health.
Department of Health (DoH) (2005a) *Everybody's Business: A Service Development Guide*. London: Department of Health.
Department of Health (DoH) (2005b) *The Mental Capacity Act (2005)*. London: Department of Health.
Department of Health (DoH) (2009) *Living Well with Dementia: A National Dementia Strategy*. London: Department of Health.
Eliopoulos, C. (2010) *Gerontological Nursing*. Philadelphia, PA. Lippincott Williams and Wilkins.

Folstein, M., Folstein, S.E. and McHugh, P.R. (1975) 'Mini Mental State' a practical method for grading the cognitive state of patients for the clinician, *Journal of Psychiatric Research*, 12(3): 189–98.

Kitwood, T. (1997) *Dementia Reconsidered*. Maidenhead: Open University Press.

Knapp, M., Thorgrimsen, L., Patel, A., Spector, A., Hallam, A., Woods, B. and Orrell, M. (2006) Cognitive stimulation therapy for people with dementia: cost effectiveness analysis, *British Journal of Psychiatry*, 188: 574–80.

Luengo-Fernandez, R., Leal, J. and Gray, A. (2010) *Dementia 2010: The Economic Burden of Dementia and Associated Research Funding in the United Kingdom*. A report produced by the Health Economics Research Centre, University of Oxford for the Alzheimer's Research Trust. Available at www.dementia2010.org.

McKeown, J., Clarke, A. and Repper, J. (2005) Life story work in health and social care: systematic literature review, *Journal of Advanced Nursing*, 55(2): 237–47.

Moniz-Cook, E. and Manthorpe, J. (eds) (2009) *Early Psychological Interventions in Dementia: Evidence-based Practice*. London: Jessica Kingsley.

National Institute for Clinical Excellence and Social Care Institute for Excellence (NICE-SCIE) (2006) *Dementia: Supporting People with Dementia and their Carers in Health and Social Care – NICE Clinical Guideline 42*. London: NICE and SCIE.

Nolan, M., Davies, S., Brown, S., Keady, J. and Nolan, J. (2004) Beyond 'person centred care': a new vision for gerontological nursing, *Journal of Clinical Nursing*, 13(9): 45–53.

Nursing and Midwifery Council (2008) *The Code: Standards of Conduct, Performance and Ethics for Nurses and Midwives*. London: Nursing and Midwifery Council.

Oyebode, J. and Clare, L. (2008) Supporting cognitive abilities, in M. Downs and B. Bowers (eds) *Excellence in Dementia Care*. Maidenhead: Open University Press.

Peters, R. (2001) The prevention of dementia, *Journal of Cardiovascular Risk*, 8: 253–6.

Roebuck, J. (1979) When does old age begin? The evolution of the English definition, *Journal of Social History*, 12(3): 416–28.

Royal College of Psychiatrists (RCP) (2009) *Factsheet: Delirium*. London: Royal College of Psychiatrists Public Education Editorial Board. Available at www.rcpsych.ac.uk (accessed 26 June 2011).

Spector, A., Thorgrimsen, L., Woods, B., Royan, L., Davies, S., Butterworth, M. and Orrell, S. (2003) Efficacy of an evidence-based cognitive stimulation therapy programme for people with dementia: randomised controlled trial, *British Journal of Psychiatry*, 183: 248–54.

Stephan, B. and Brayne, C. (2008) Prevalence and projections of dementia, in M. Downs and B. Bowers (eds) *Excellence in Dementia Care*. Maidenhead: Open University Press.

World Health Organization (WHO) (1993a) *The ICD-10 Classification of Mental and Behavioural Disorders: Diagnostic Criteria for Research*. Geneva: WHO.

World Health Organization (WHO) (1993b) *The ICD-10 Classification of Mental and Behavioural Disorders: Clinical Descriptions and Diagnostic Guidelines*. Geneva: WHO.

World Health Organization (2003) *International Statistical Classification of Diseases and Related Health Problems: 10th Revision Version*. Geneva: WHO.

10 Psychological interventions and working with children and adolescents

John Harrison

Chapter aim and objectives

Aim
- The aim of this chapter is to introduce the reader to the specific needs of children and adolescents in terms of psychological interventions.

Objectives
- To provide a brief introduction to the concept of cognitive development and its part in diagnosis and treatment within mental health.
- To discuss the particular 'tiered' approach to treatment for young people suffering mental ill health within the UK.
- To introduce art therapy as a psychological intervention for young people.
- To introduce play therapy as a psychological intervention for young people.

An introduction to working with children and adolescents

This chapter, like others in the book, will examine some of the psychological interventions that are available in the treatment of mental ill health. However, it will do so while considering a number of important factors. First, cognitive ability as well as the physical age of the young person will always need to be considered before a diagnosis can be given and treatment commenced. Therefore, the impact of what is deemed appropriate psychological functioning will be discussed before the psychological interventions are introduced. Second, the approach to the treatment of mental illness in the young differs a great deal from that offered to adults.

Child and Adolescent Mental Health Services (CAMHS) provide a unique tier system in the treatment of psychological ill health in the young (Royal College of Psychiatrists, 2008). Nurses are among a range of professionals providing specialist treatment in a range of settings. As well as some of the psychological therapies discussed in other chapters of this book, there are two approaches that have a particular place within CAMHS, namely art and play therapy. It is an exploration of psychological interventions framed within these specific two approaches that will form the bulk of this chapter and, as such, its appearance will differ from what is the norm in the rest of the book (Department of Health, 2006b; Nursing and Midwifery Council, 2010).

There is not space within this chapter to discuss the subject of child development in depth, and further reading will provide a greater understanding of why development plays such an important part in the treatments designed for children and young people (Black and Cottrell, 1993). In essence, the issue is one of age: what would be considered normal psychological functioning for one age group of children would be seen as an indication of mental ill health in another (Hughes and Graham, 2002). For example, the imaginary role-play acted out by very young children is a vital element in their psychosocial development as they make use of play to understand the world around them (Landreth, 2002). As such, it is quite common for younger children to allow some of this imagery into the 'real world', often perceiving everyday objects as having imaginary power or abilities. Similar behaviours in an adolescent would suggest that there is a mental health issue that needs to be addressed. Therefore, age and cognition play a central part in developing an understanding of how psychological problems can be identified and treated (Barker, 1995). For the purpose of this chapter, a young person will mean anyone under the age of 18 at the time of treatment.

Another issue to consider is that childhood is a time of change, both physically and socially. As such, events like starting school, parental separation and adolescence can have a huge impact on a young person's mental well-being (Hughes and Graham, 2002). Thus, conditions such as anxiety disorder have been identified as common among young people (Khanna and Kendall, 2010). But, what is important is not that the conditions themselves cause problems for the young person, it is how they impact on the important issue of education. It is long established that school not only pro-vides an education in terms of academic subjects, but also plays a vital role in our psy-chosocial development as we move into adulthood (Dadds and Barrett, 2001). Many psychological interventions are therefore aimed at ensuring that, as much as possible, the young person can remain in full-time education (Axelrad et al., 2009). This policy of as little intervention and disruption as needed is central to the tier system used in CAMHS.

The mental health services that have been developed for children and young peo-ple within the UK provide a unique treatment system. As emphasis was increasingly placed on providing a service for children that met their needs, the NHS Health Advi-sory Service published the review *Together We Stand* (1995). This document established the four-tier system model of treatment as a national approach to child mental illness. Each tier is seen as providing care of an increasingly specialised nature (McDougall et al., 2008).

> Tier one: This is the initial stage of the CAMHS process. As such the majority of staff are not mental health professionals but are often those who come into regular contact with the young person, such as teachers and youth workers. The role here is one of minor intervention and health promotion, although referral to and working alongside other services is common (Charman, 2004).
> Tier two: This second stage may be the young person's first contact with special-ist mental health practitioners. Based in community settings, though often

working independently, they include therapists, paediatricians and primary mental health workers. These staff are often involved in dealing with children who present with emotional and behavioural problems in school settings (Axelrad et al., 2009).

- Tier three: This tier is characterized by groups of child mental health specialists often working in multidisciplinary settings. These include psychologists, specialist nurses and child psychiatrists. Emphasis is on community-based treatments that may require more long-term or specialised input than that found in the earlier tiers. Therapies such as art and play therapy are often utilized at this level.
- Tier four: These are highly specialized services based around in-patient treatment. Often treatments involve intense and multi-approach therapies for children and young people suffering from complex, severe and long-term mental illness (McDougall et al., 2008). Alongside a range of treatment approaches, including pharmacological intervention, use is made of a range of psychological interventions ranging from art and play therapies through to complex family therapies lasting many months (Cotterall and Kraam, 2005). Tier-four treatment is often residential in nature and may include secure environments for those who are considered to be a risk to themselves or others (Jaffa et al., 2004).

While these tiers suggest a level of progression, this is only in terms of complexity of treatment. A patient does not necessarily move through each of the tiers in turn and can move from the care team in tier one to tier four and back again in the course of their treatment. The tiers are also not exclusive of one another, and it is common for a young person to receive support from professionals from across a number of tiers as a package of care and treatment is developed. This complex approach to care is underpinned by the concept of 'in the child's best interest', which balances the rights of the young person and their family to freedom of action with the equal rights of treatment and safety.

Risk, in terms of psychological interventions involving young people, often comes down to issues of conflict (also see Chapter 1). There may be a conflict between confidentiality and patient safety or the knowledge that long-term treatment may result in the loss of important educational chances. Throughout all this, those providing care must work in the 'best interests' of the child as established in the Department of Health guidelines (DoH, 2004). As such, clinicians must balance issues of boundaries and confidentiality with risk management, listening to the concerns of the young person and taking what they have to say seriously (also see Chapter 11) (Sondheimer, 2010).

Art therapy and scenario

Art is an integral part of human existence and has been used by us to express our fears and desires since the earliest societies (Biley and Galvin, 2007). Art itself can be seen as a therapeutic experience, allowing us to make use of the creative nature that exists within each of us. Both Freud and Jung believed that art was a means of expressing the inner self (Malchiodi, 2006). Art therapy has grown, in part, out of this idea. It is used as a means of communication, whereby the individual is able to use art to express their inner experiences and beliefs through the creation of an art work (Malchiodi, 2003). The aim of the art therapy session is to allow the patient to make sense of their experiences, while being guided and supported by the therapist. This is particularly relevant when the expression of feelings verbally may be particularly difficult (Pretorius and Pfifer, 2010).

The art therapist is trained to facilitate the individual in teasing out what the art represents. The therapist then explores the hidden metaphors and meanings within the art and what it is that the individual is saying within their art work (Malchiodi, 2006). The therapist does not interpret what has been produced in isolation but explores the art work in context, allowing the patient to provide meaning to their work. Use is made of a range of materials, from paints and pencils through to the use of clay for modelling and in some cases photography, depending on the age and cognitive abilities of the patients as well as the nature and severity of their condition (Case and Dalley, 2007).

Although not a medium developed exclusively for the young, the use of art therapy with children has been well established (Manicom and Boronska, 2003; Epp, 2008). Its use within diagnosis and treatment began with the psychologist Florence Goodenough, who several decades ago created the 'draw a man test' as a means of measuring a child's intelligence. The more complex the drawing, the greater the potential academic ability of the child. The use of art as a means of dealing with psychological issues has become increasingly established within the clinical environment. As such, art therapists are regulated by their own professional body and are now accepted as an integral part of the multidisciplinary team. Art is seen as an activity that children enjoy and find acceptable (Epp, 2008). Children are able to use art to develop a sense of control and competence as well as developing an understanding of the world around them, often drawing objects that are familiar and important to them, such as parents (Simard and Nielsen, 2009). The use of art in therapy stems from this sense of security; some clinicians suggest that some children may feel overawed by verbalizing their experiences to others and may prefer using art as a medium in which to explore their experiences and emotions (Pretorius and Pfifer, 2010).

Others feel that art therapy acknowledges the cognitive functioning of very young people, who may have difficulty in verbalizing their feelings. As such, psychological interventions that are used with adults would not be suitable (Zehnder et al., 2010). Therefore, the child may make use of art as a medium for disclosing painful events, providing images that allow for the detection of psychological problems (Blain et al., 1981; Malchiodi, 1997).

In order to understand how art therapies are used by clinicians, two of the more established methods, 'House, Tree, Person' and the Diagnostic Drawing Series, will be explored. Each of these approaches follows a set pattern and will allow for a greater insight into how art therapy allows for the emotions of the young person to emerge.

Developed in 1982 by Cohen and Lesowitz, the 'House, Tree, Person' method is often used in work with adolescents within in-patient environments as part of an overall psychiatric assessment involving a range of clinicians including nursing staff. The patient is invited to first draw any picture, making use of any colour they wish.

They are then asked to draw a tree and finally asked to use any colour or shape that they wish in order to draw how they are feeling. The role of the therapist is then to interpret what each of the drawings means. The first drawing is meant to represent the patient's defence mechanisms. The tree is designed to be an insight into the patient's psychic state or level of mental functioning. The final drawing is intended to show how the patient is feeling. The types of shape drawn and the colours used by the patient are then rated according to a diagnostic checklist and alongside a psychiatric assessment, to provide a picture of the young person's mental health (Brooke, 2004).

Based on a psychoanalytical concept by Buck (1966), the drawings are meant to provide an insight into the subconscious of the patient and, as such, give insight into how they are functioning psychologically when they are compared against a scoring system based on feelings and self-perception. Again, the young person is asked to draw three images (a house, a tree and a person), all of which are seen as a reflection of the self. As they do so the therapist asks a number of questions.

As the young person draws the house they are asked such questions as: who lives there? What goes on inside? What happens at night? Does anyone visit? Alongside the questions asked by the therapist, the drawing itself is open for interpretation. For instance, small windows and doors can be seen as demonstrating insecurity on the part of the patient. While the tree is drawn, the therapist then asks questions such as: What type of tree is it? How old is the tree? What goes on nearby? Has anyone tried to cut the tree down? The drawing itself is providing an indication of the how the person feels about themselves: large and out-reaching branches are felt to indicate the patients wish to achieve something, while drawing roots shows that they feel grounded and secure within themselves.

The drawing of the person provides the therapist with the chance to ask how the young person feels about themselves. Questions include: who is the person in the picture? What do they enjoy doing? Who cares for them? Has anyone tried to hurt them? Lack of detail within the drawing, an incomplete drawing or one that is done only faintly are felt to be indicators of withdrawal or depression as are expressions of sadness or tearfulness on the face of the image (Malchiodi, 2003).

The clinical environments in which such techniques can be used are numerous. Art therapy has been used to deal with the psychological impact of sexual and physical abuse (Pretorius and Pfifer, 2010) as well as dealing with the trauma of events such as natural disasters and road traffic accidents. In such cases, it is felt that the use of art allows the patient to provide a narrative of events. These narratives allow the patient to explore what has taken place and attempt to confront and then come to terms with painful memories and look for ways of moving forward (Simard and Neilsen, 2009). Other uses include work done with young people with eating disorders. Art allows the patient to develop a sense of self through what they create. Once this has been established, the art work is then used to develop relationships with others, particularly the therapist, in what becomes a shared experience. This allows for anxieties to be discussed and addressed through a safe and comfortable medium (Case and Dalley, 2007). In some cases, therapy sessions can be spread over a number of weeks, though there are instances of early intervention, single-session treatments being of benefit to children involved in road traffic accidents (RTAs), as the following scenario demonstrates.

SCENARIO

Ten-year-old Harriet is brought into the clinic by her parents after a referral from her general practitioner. Five days earlier both Harriet and her mother had been involved in an RTA and, although not physically injured, both were badly shaken by what took place. Since the accident took place Harriet has been showing signs of anxiety around the event. Normally a happy, confident child, she has become tearful, particularly when either of her parents leaves the house, expressing the fear that they may be involved in another RTA and becoming unwilling to sleep until everyone is back within the family home. When her parents have tried to comfort her, she becomes unwilling to discuss what has happened.

At the clinic, Harriet is introduced to Charlotte, an art therapist. Charlotte then follows a four-stage programme making use of art to facilitate the process. First, she asks Harriet to reconstruct what happened by drawing the RTA in order to aid the therapeutic dialogue. Harriet is then asked what her thoughts are of the event. When she describes the trauma of the accident and expresses her anxieties since, Charlotte is able discuss alternatives, pointing out that such events are rare and that Harriet should not worry about her parents being in cars any more than she did before.

This is done to identify any dysfunctional appraisal the patient has of the event and to attempt to modify them. Finally, Charlotte is able to tell Harriet that her feelings are perfectly understandable and that most people will have some degree of anxiety. This helps to normalize the emotions that Harriet has towards the RTA. The session ends with Charlotte discussing the outcome with both Harriet and her parents. Charlotte explains the importance of a daily routine and talking about the event as a family to help keep symptoms to a minimum, and a leaflet is provided offering information on childhood anxiety and details of further support where needed. After the session, Harriet and her parents were able to talk about what had happened and how some of what Charlotte has said has made her feel less anxious.

The chance to observe art therapy in action is often open to those who find themselves on placement with CAMHS teams. Student nurses should be encouraged to explore how art therapy is used in conjunction with other therapies (Department of Health, 2006a; 2006b; Nursing and Midwifery Council, 2010). Discuss with members of the CAMHS team how they use art therapy and how the age of the patient plays an important part in its implementation.

Play therapy and scenario

Although art therapy is a unique therapeutic approach in its own right, there is another psychological therapy that makes use of drawing in its treatment for young people with mental health issues. Play therapy has its roots in Freudian psychoanalysis and is based around the concept of the 'therapeutic power of play' (Ledyard, 1999).

Play is an essential and natural part of a child's psychosocial development. Through play, children are able to develop problem-solving skills and learn to deal with social interaction and the creation of rules. As a result, play is felt to help develop a strong sense of self and to aid self-confidence (Siu, 2010). Given the importance of play in the life of young people, the development of a therapeutic intervention based on the act of playing would seem natural (Cochran et al., 2010). What has emerged as a result of this belief is the concept of play therapy. As we shall see, there is a range of therapeutic approaches that have play as their central feature. Each places an emphasis on a different aspect of what play therapy is and how it benefits the young person, but a working definition of what takes place is given by Webb (2007: 46): 'Play therapy is a helping interaction between trained adult therapists and a child for the purpose of relieving the child's emotional distress by using the symbolic communication of play.'

As the definition indicates, play therapy is often utilized for the treatment of psychological issues in the younger patient. Although its use has been found in dealing with mental illness among the elderly (Ledyard, 1999), emphasis is placed on the way play is perceived by children. Before the age of 7, play is not make believe for most children but is a vital part of their subjective reality (Dougherty and Ray, 2007). Therefore, any intervention that uses play as a medium has a real chance of making vast improvements in a child's psychological functioning (Nichols, 2010).

As play therapy has developed as a method of treatment, its clinical uses have diverged, resulting in a number of different approaches. As with art therapy, specially trained therapists (which include nursing staff and teachers) adopt a range of skills to overcome a number of psychological problems. These methods range from the treatment of long-standing psychosocial dysfunction (Muro et al., 2006) to the issue of anxieties prior to hospital admission (Siu, 2010). Often used in conjunction with other psychological therapies, such as family therapy (Bowers, 2009), play therapy can essentially be divided into two distinct groups, directive and non-directive. In essence, these differences are based around how the therapeutic sessions are developed. In non-directive therapy, the patient is allowed to suggest the play activity and help in the establishment of ground rules. In directive therapy, the therapist decides on the structure of the play and sets limits on behaviour (Webb, 2007).

Whichever approach is taken, emphasis is placed on play as a means of communication. For many young people, expressing their concerns and anxieties can be a problem. This is especially the case for younger children, who may lack the ability to verbalize what they are experiencing (Muro et al., 2006). Through play, the patient is able to express their emotions and think through what they have experienced. Therapy often takes place within a designated playroom, in which the child learns to feel secure and able to interact without fear of judgement (Nichols, 2010). Use is made of a range of equipment in order to aid the session, including puppets, miniature figures and sandpits in which the child is able to act out what is concerning them without having to verbalize their fears (Nims, 2007). The role of the therapist is to interact with the patient through the act of play, offer a listening ear and in later sessions help formulate solutions that may help overcome the problem. This can take the form of role-play using puppets, in which the patient is able to re-create hurtful events or discuss concerns via the cathartic nature of play (Webb, 2007). Labels are given to the problem, not the child, and this helps externalize the issue, making it easier to develop strategies in the form of cognitive behavioural therapy or solution-focused brief therapy (Nims, 2007;

Nichols, 2010). Often therapy can last over a period of many weeks and for as many as 24 individual sessions (Bowers, 2009).

This process of the child becoming at ease with the environment, discussing issues through play and finding solutions is best described in the system offered by Lantz and Raiz (2003).

1   *Holding:* the first stage of therapy, this allows the child to bring repressed emotions and feelings into the open within the safe, accepting environment of the play room.
2   *Telling:* the child is able to disclose what has taken place or describe their pain and anxiety. Issues cease to be an internal problem and become something that can be shared in an effective and therapeutic way.
3   *Mastering:* once the issue has been discussed, the child and therapist look at solutions that will allow the issue to be overcome in a constructive and forward-moving way.
4   *Honouring:* finding ways of making something positive out of the experience.

The following scenario will explore how play therapists make use of materials such as puppets in order to aid the healing process for younger children.

SCENARIO

Jemima, aged 7, has been referred to a play therapist after her parents expressed concerns around her withdrawn and sullen behaviour. Sally, the play therapist, introduces Jemima to a range of glove puppets and over a number of sessions she is able to give each a name and construct a narrative about them, naming one of the puppets Emily, who she says is a girl of the same age. Sally notes that, while playing, Jemima often talks of the sadness that the puppets feel. As the sessions progress, Jemima is able to say that the sadness felt by the puppets is caused by the loss of someone they care about. Sally discusses this with Jemima's parents who inform her that six months before the therapy began Jemima's uncle had died. This had affected the family greatly and as it caused both parents a great deal of distress it was not something that was discussed. Sally was able through the play sessions to discover if this too had happened to Emily and what could be done to make the sadness go away. Together, Jemima and Sally are able to look at ways in which Emily can feel better while still remembering the person she had lost, saying that it is normal for people to feel sad if someone they love dies and that the person Emily lost would not wish her to be sad for ever. The solutions came through the act of play, with Jemima being able to develop the scenarios in which things could be improved. Throughout the process, Sally offers solutions and is able to draw Jemima towards some constructive conclusions of her own. As the sessions draw to a close, Jemima's parents state that she is far less withdrawn and that they have been able to discuss the death of her uncle as a family. Sally and Jemima look at ways in which her uncle can be remembered, Jemima deciding that she would plant a tree for her uncle in her back garden with the help of her parents, stating that she felt Emily would do the same.

There is increasing use of play therapy within the framework of CAMHS as the government aims to improve mental health and well-being among the young (McDougall, 2011). If you are placed in an environment in which play therapy is used, take the chance to discuss its benefits with clinicians. Spending time with younger patients and engaging with them in appropriate forms of play is part of the therapeutic process and you should reflect on how this shapes your understanding of how young people construct their understanding of the world (Department of Health, 2006a; 2006b; Nursing and Midwifery Council, 2010).

Summary of the key points

Childhood and adolescence offer particular challenges to those working with young people suffering from psychological problems.
In order to facilitate treatment, mental health services have been developed especially for the young, in a system different to that offered to adults.
The nature of working with the young offers some particular issues in terms of risk that the mental health nurse should be aware of.
The issue of cognitive development means that there are some treatments such as art and play therapies that work particularly well with the young.
Both art and play therapies are often used in conjunction with other treatments.

Quick quiz

1   How does age differ from cognitive development?
2   How many tiers of treatment are there in a CAMHS?
3   At which stage of the tier system will in-patient provision be made?
4   Why is it necessary to develop treatments that are age particular for younger children?
5   How does art therapy aid in the disclosure of painful experiences for young people?
6   How can aids such as puppets help the play therapist engage in treatment with younger clients?
7   In what way does directive play therapy differ from non-directive play?

References

Axelrad, M., Garland, B. and Love, K. (2009) Brief behavioural interventions for young children with disruptive behaviours, *Journal of Clinical Psychology in Medical Settings*, 16: 263–9.
Barker, P. (1995) *Basic Child Psychiatry*. London, Blackwell.
Biley, F. and Galvin, K. (2007) Lifeworld, the arts and mental health nursing, *Journal of Psychiatric and Mental Health Nursing*, 14: 800–7.
Black, D. and Cottrell, D. (1993) *Seminars in Child and Adolescent Psychiatry*. London: Gaskill.

Blain, G., Bergner, R., Lewis, M. and Goldstein, M. (1981) The use of objectively scorable house – tree – person indicators to establish child abuse, *Journal of Clinical Psychology*, 3: 667–73.

Bowers, N. (2009) A naturalistic study of the early relationship development process of nondirective play therapy, *International Journal of Play Therapy*, 3: 176–89.

Brooke, L. (2004) *Tools of the Trade: A Therapist's Guide to Art Therapy Assessments*. Springfield, IL: Charles C. Thomas.

Buck, J. (1966) *The House–Tree–Person Technique: Revised Manual*. Los Angeles, CA: Western Psychological Services.

Case, C. and Dalley, T. (eds) (2007) *Art Therapy with Children: From Infancy to Adolescence*. London: Routledge.

Charman, S. (2004) Mental health services for children and young people: the past, present and future of service development and policy, *Mental Health Review*, 9: 6–14.

Cochran, J., Fauth, D., Cochran, N., Spurgeon, S. and Pierce, L. (2010) Growing play therapy up: extending child-centred play therapy to highly aggressive teenage boys, *Person-centred and Experiential Psychotherapies*, 9: 292–300.

Cotterall, D. and Kraam, A. (2005) Growing up? A history of CAMHS (1987–2005), *Child and Adolescent Mental Health*, 10: 111–17.

Dadds, M. and Barrett, P. (2001) Practitioner review: psychological management of anxiety disorders in childhood, *Journal of Child Psychology and Psychiatry*, 8: 999–1011.

Department of Health (DoH) (2004) *National Service Framework for Children, Young People and Maternity Services: The Mental Health and Psychological Well Being of Children and Young People*. London: Stationery Office.

Department of Health (DoH) (2006a) *From Values to Action: The Chief Nursing Officer's Review of Mental Health Nursing*. London: Department of Health.

Department of Health (DoH) (2006b) *Best Practice Competencies and Capabilities for Pre-registration Mental Health Nurses in England: The Chief Nursing Officer's Review of Mental Health Nursing*. London: Department of Health.

Dougherty, J. and Ray, D. (2007) Differential impact of play therapy on developmental levels of children, *International Journal of Play Therapy*, 1: 2–19.

Epp, K. (2008) Outcome-based evaluation of a social skills program using art therapy and group therapy for children on the autism spectrum, *Children and Schools*, 30: 27–36.

Hughes, C. and Graham, A. (2002) Measuring executive functions in childhood: problems and solutions, *Child and Adolescent Mental Health*, 7: 131–43.

Jaffa, T., Lelliott, P., O'Herlihy, A., Worrall, A., Hill, P. and Banerjee, S. (2004) The staffing of inpatient child and adolescent mental health services, *Child and Adolescent Mental Health*, 9: 84–7.

Khanna, M. and Kendall, P. (2010) Computer assisted cognitive behavioural therapy for child anxiety: results of a randomised clinical trail, *Journal of Consulting and Clinical Psychology*, 78: 737–45.

Landreth, G. (2002) *Play Therapy: The Art of the Relationship*, 2nd edn. New York: Routledge.

Lantz, J. and Raiz, L. (2003) Play and art in existential trauma therapy with children and their parents, *Contemporary Family Therapy*, 25: 165–77.

Ledyard, P. (1999) Play therapy with the elderly: a case study, *International Journal of Play Therapy*, 2: 57–75.

McDougall, T. (2011) Improving mental health outcomes for children and young people, *Mental Health Practice*, 14: 22–4.

Malchiodi, C. (1997) *Breaking the Silence: Art Therapy with Children from Violent Homes.* London: Psychology Press.

Malchiodi, C. (ed.) (2003) *Handbook of Art Therapy.* New York: Guilford Press.

Malchiodi, C. (2006) *The Art Therapy Sourcebook.* New York: McGraw-Hill.

Manicom, H. and Boronska, T. (2003) Co-creating change within a child protection system: integrating art therapy with family therapy practice, *Journal of Family Therapy*, 25: 217–32.

McDougall, T., Worral-Davies, A., Hewson, L., Richardson, G. and Cotgrove, A. (2008) Tier 4 Child and Adolescent Mental Health Services (CAMHS) – inpatient care day services and alternatives: an overview of tier 4 CAMHS provision in the UK, *Child and Adolescent Mental Health*, 4: 173–80.

Muro, J., Ray, D., Schottlkorb, A. and Smith, M. (2006) Quantitative analysis of long-term child centred play therapy, *International Journal of Play Therapy*, 15: 35–58.

NHS Health Advisory Service (1995) *Together We Stand: Thematic Review of the Commissioning, Role and Management of Child and Adolescent Mental Health Services.* London: HMSO.

Nichols, J. (2010) Assisting anxious children, *Kai Tiaki Nursing New Zealand*, 16: 12–14.

Nims, D. (2007) Integrating play therapy techniques into solution-focused brief therapy, *International Journal of Play Therapy*, 1: 54–68.

Nursing and Midwifery Council (2010) *Standards for Pre-registration Nursing Education.* London: Nursing and Midwifery Council.

Pretorius, G. and Pfifer, N. (2010) Group art therapy with sexually abused girls, *South African Journal of Psychology*, 40: 63–73.

Royal College of Psychiatrists (2008) *Child and Adolescent Psychiatrists: How They Can Help.* London: Royal College of Psychiatrists.

Simard, V. and Nielsen, T. (2009) Adaptation of imagery rehearsal therapy for nightmares in children: a brief report, *Psychotherapy Theory, Research, Practice, Training*, 46: 492–7.

Siu, A. (2010) Play therapy in Hong Kong: opportunities and challenges, *International Journal of Play Therapy*, 4: 235–43.

Sondheimer, A. (2010) Ethics and risk management in administrative child and adolescent psychiatry, *Child and Adolescent Psychiatric Clinics of North America*, 19: 115–29.

Webb, N. (ed.) (2007) *Play Therapy with Children in Crisis: Individual, Group and Family Treatment.* New York: Guilford Press.

Zehnder, D., Meuli, M. and Landolt, M. (2010) Effectiveness of a single session early psychological intervention for children after road traffic accidents: a randomised controlled trial, *Child and Adolescent Psychiatry and Mental Health*, 4: 1–10.

11 Psychological interventions within an ethical context

Grahame Smith

Chapter aim and objectives

Aim

- To explore psychological interventions within an ethical reasoning context.

Objectives

- To describe relevant and key ethical theories.
- To identify how professional rules are used.
- To apply an ethically reasoned approach.
- To consider the use of a values-based practice approach.
- To analyse the impact of power as an ethical issue.

Introduction

The aim of this chapter is to explore and consider within a mental health nursing context the potential ethical issues that may arise from the use of psychological interventions. This chapter will not specifically address the legal context of mental health nursing, but it is recommended as part of the ongoing development of your ethical reasoning skills that you avail yourself of a good mental health law text. The mental health nurse, as the identified professional within the therapeutic relationship, will be expected to act ethically and do the 'right thing' (Roberts, 2004; Department of Health, 2006a; 2006b; O'Carroll and Park, 2007; Nursing and Midwifery Council, 2008; Warne et al., 2011). Knowing how to act ethically is based on the mental health nurse being able to utilize the relevant ethical theories, understand the relevant professional rules, and also having the skills to ethically reason; on this basis the intention of this chapter will be to explore these three tenets in greater detail (Roberts, 2004; Thompson et al., 2006).

It is also important to recognize that acting ethically within a mental health nursing context has to account for the value-laden nature of mental health nursing. This means that during the process of ethically reasoning the mental health nurse cannot just rely on a rules-based approach to solve the issue at hand (Roberts, 2004; Callaghan, 2009; Fulford, 2009; Warne et al., 2011). That is not to say that rules-based approaches are not helpful or that mental health nurses should not follow them, but there certainly is a need to complement these approaches by considering the role of values. 'The recent Chief Nursing Officer's review of mental health nursing in England, From Values to Action (DH, 2006[a]), and the Scottish Review of Mental Health Nursing, Rights, Relationships and Recovery (Scottish Executive, 2006), both emphasize the important role of values in mental health nursing' (Cooper, 2009: 25).

On the basis that the mental health nurse has to robustly consider the role of values, this chapter will explore how this can be achieved by considering the work of Woodbridge and Fulford (2004). It is also important to note that mental health nursing practice has a controlling element, whereby the mental health nurse doing good may also mean they have to restrict freedoms (Roberts, 2004; 2005; Callaghan, 2009; Mitchell, 2011). The downside of the power to control is that the potential to intentionally or unintentionally abuse this power is an ever present concern. On this basis the chapter will consider how the mental health nurse can ethically navigate through this concern (Borthwick et al., 2001; Roberts, 2004; Chodoff, 2009; Mitchell, 2011).

To ensure that the ideas, notions and concepts considered in this chapter have a practical value the following scenario will be used and developed throughout the chapter.

SCENARIO

Anne has been admitted informally to an acute mental health ward; this is Anne's first admission. The circumstances leading up to the admission relate to Anne taking 40 paracetamol tablets with the clear intention of killing herself (expressed by Anne on interview) and ending what Anne calls her 12 months of 'suffering and despair'. Anne was provisionally diagnosed as having depression (severe). As Anne still felt 'suicidal' it was decided to arrange a short admission with the aim of devising a comprehensive care package tailored to her needs.

Ethical theory

In order for the mental health nurse to act ethically when delivering psychological interventions they have to be able to ethically reason in a way that utilizes the relevant ethical theory. Mental health nurses who ethically reason in this way have an advantage in that the chosen course of action will be based on critically analysing the strengths and limitations of any ethical theory relevant to the situation (Bloch and Green, 2009; Barker 2011). Bearing this in mind, the aim of this section is to assist the mental health nurse in their journey of understanding ethical theory by providing a whistlestop tour of the major ethical theories prevalent within a mental health context.

Generally, ethical theories can be divided into normative and non-normative theories. Normative ethical theories focus on what actions are right, what ought to be done, what motives are good and what characteristics are virtuous (Beauchamp and Childress, 2009; Barker 2011). Non-normative theories focus on understanding people's ethical beliefs and conduct and how they ethically reason. Unlike normative ethics, non-normative ethics is not interested in prescribing such things as what action is right or not right (Sumner, 1967; Beauchamp and Childress, 2009; Barker 2011). For the purposes of this chapter we will concentrate on ethical theories which are normative theories.

Historically, two ethical theories have dominated normative ethics: consequentialism and deontology. Not only have these two ethical theories been dominant, but in the process of countering these theories other ethical theories have emerged (LaFollette, 2000).

Consequentialism, also known as utilitarianism, generally takes the view that determining whether an action is ethical or not ethical is based on the outcome of that action: the implication for the mental health nurse is that to be ethical their actions should 'produce the greatest balance of good over bad' (LaFollette, 2000; Bloch and Green, 2009). Using the chapter scenario as an example, admitting Anne to an acute mental health ward as a way of managing risk and reducing harms (a good thing) could be seen as ethical if it prevents Anne from harming herself. However, it could be seen as unethical (a bad thing) if it leads to Anne harming herself again. A difficulty with this approach is finding an agreed way to accurately calculate whether a particular action led to a particular outcome. For instance, if Anne did harm herself after being admitted to the ward, the majority of the parties involved, and after excluding all other possible causes, would have to agree that Anne harming herself did, indeed, occur as a direct consequence of being admitted to the ward (Bloch and Green, 2009).

Deontology in its purest form, or the 'study of duty' (also known as 'Kantianism'), takes the general stance that, based on reason, the ethical person without exception must always do their duty (LaFollette, 2000; Seedhouse, 2009). Returning to the chapter scenario, according to a deontological approach the mental health nurse's ethical duty would be to prevent Anne from committing suicide. A problem with the deontological approach occurs when two or more duties conflict. For example the mental health nurse has a duty to Anne to respect her capacity for self-determination but also has a duty to prevent Anne from committing suicide. This potentially puts the nurse in the situation where they have to choose one ethical duty over another (Bloch and Green, 2009).

Consequentialism and deontology are at times dominant ethical theories, but within the context of mental health care there are also a number of other ethical theories which need to be mentioned such as virtue ethics, care ethics and principlism (Bloch and Green, 2009; Edwards, 2009; Barker 2011).

Virtue ethics takes the broad view that being ethical is based on the character of a person. A virtuous person will therefore acquire traits such as honesty, trustworthiness, cooperativeness and humility, will contribute to virtuous behaviour and, in turn, live ethically (Smith and Godfrey, 2002). Within the scenario the mental health nurse would utilize their character traits to not only emotionally respond to Anne and her situation, but also to guide their ethical reasoning. For example, preventing Anne from committing suicide is not just about deciding it is wrong, the nurse has to also use such character traits as being trustworthy, motivated and empathic to help Anne manage this risky behaviour (McKie and Swinton, 2000; Roberts, 2004). A key difficulty with a virtue ethics approach is that there is a lack of consensus about which traits are an essential part of being virtuous and also on how virtuous traits are acquired (Bloch and Green, 2009).

Care ethics, which can be seen to draw on virtue theory, developmental psychology, feminist thinking and the work of the Scottish philosopher Dave Hume, values the extending of care to vulnerable people, with the emphasis on compassion (Bloch and Green, 2009; Horsfield et al., 2011). In terms of the scenario, the mental health nurse will utilize the therapeutic relationship as a way of being ethical. The nurse will utilize virtuous traits described above but they will also consider that managing Anne's risky behaviour has to also take into account Anne's perspective, such as what Anne wants, and how this would relate to Anne being part of a social network (Roberts, 2004; Horsfield et al., 2011). The difficulty with this approach is similar to the difficulty of applying a virtue ethics approach, with the added problem of this approach being relative to the situation. Therefore, the nurse may find that an ethical solution for one situation is not necessarily applicable to another, albeit similar, situation (Bloch and Green, 2009; Horsfield et al., 2011).

Principlism is, as the name suggests, based on using principles in moral decision-making. The principles are: do no harm (non-maleficence); act to benefit others (beneficence); respect a person's autonomy; and treat people fairly (justice) (Roberts, 2004; Bloch and Green, 2009; Barker 2011). In relation to Anne's situation there appear, in the first instance, to be two principles that have to be considered: beneficence, that is benefiting Anne by preventing her from committing suicide; and respecting Anne's autonomy by taking into account her right to determine her life. These principles also appear to conflict. Does the nurse allow Anne to commit suicide, thereby breaching the principle of beneficence, or does the nurse stop Anne from committing suicide, thereby potentially breaching the principle of respect for autonomy. Beauchamp and Childress (2009) suggest that where there is a conflict of principles a further level of analysis needs to take place, where all factors are taken into account. In this case Anne is diagnosed with a mental illness, and if she is deemed not to be acting autonomously (lacks capacity) the principle of respect for autonomy does not need to be considered to be as important as the principle of beneficence. On this basis the nurse is obligated to intervene and prevent Anne from committing suicide. The major difficulty with the four-principle approach compared with any other ethical theory and according to Seedhouse (2009: 99) 'is that it does not explain why one should follow it'.

In the next section we will look at how moral theories combined with professional codes work as part of the ethical reasoning process.

Ethical practice, guidelines and reasoning

When utilizing psychological interventions mental health nurses require specific knowledge and skills, however there is also the professional expectation that they will follow specific ethical rules (including any relevant legal frameworks) and exhibit certain values and behaviours (Callaghan, 2009; Mitchell, 2011). For the purposes of this chapter, though, we are looking at psychological interventions within a mental health nursing context. It is important to note that although mental health nursing is professionally aligned to the nursing community, historically and politically it has also been heavily influenced by other professional disciplines such as psychiatry and psychology (Department of Health, 2006a; 2006b; Callaghan, 2009). The potential impact at a practice level is that the mental health nurse would ordinarily locate themselves within the professional community of nursing which would involve following the relevant ethical code; but for some mental health nurses, who, at the same time, work as therapists, they may also need to consider other relevant professional codes (Coady, 2009).

As previously stated we will be focusing on psychological interventions within a mental health nursing context and on that basis the professional body for nursing is the Nursing and Midwifery Council (NMC) which describes itself thus:

- We exist to safeguard the health and wellbeing of the public.
- We set the standards of education, training and conduct that nurses and midwives need to deliver high quality healthcare consistently throughout their careers.
- We ensure that nurses and midwives keep their skills and knowledge up to date and uphold the standards of their professional code.
- We ensure that midwives are safe to practise by setting rules for their practice and supervision.
- We have fair processes to investigate allegations made against nurses and midwives who may not have followed the code.

(NMC, 2008: 1)

Like most professional bodies the NMC requires mental health nurses to follow a professional code which, in this instance, takes the form of a code of conduct based on four ethical statements:

1 Make the care of people your first concern, treating them as individuals and respecting their dignity
2 Work with others to protect and promote health and wellbeing of those in your care, their families and carers, and the wider community
3 Provide a high standard of practice and care at all times
4 Be open and honest, act with integrity and uphold the reputation of the profession.

(NMC, 2008: 2)

The aim of any professional code, including the NMC's, is to establish standards of professional conduct and, in doing so it also offers behavioural guidelines, that is how the professional should or should not act (Ford, 2006; NMC, 2008). This guidance is usually generalized, for example the NMC's (2008: 6) ethical statement, 'provide a high standard of practice and care at all times', guides the mental health nurse to consider that using best evidence within their practice is a good thing to do. It does not, however, and nor does it intend to, give you specific detail on what should be done in every given situation. The code does not provide the mental health nurse with a specific method of resolving ethical dilemmas. Rather it gives the nurse a framework to work within, and on that basis the nurse working within this framework must also develop their own ability to ethically reason (Ford, 2006; Nursing and Midwifery Council, 2010).

Developing the ability to ethically reason is a skill which requires the mental health nurse to, first, identify the ethical issues at hand and, second, to critically reflect on those identified issues (Fulford et al., 2006). Certainly, recognizing and reflecting on an ethical issue is an important first step in the process, but for this process to be something that the mental health nurse can learn from it needs to also be rational and systematic (Ford, 2006). If we consider the chapter scenario there are number of ethical issues that can be identified. The key issue that we will concentrate on is that acute mental health wards can intentionally or unintentionally restrict certain freedoms (Roberts, 2004; Horsfield et al., 2011). Based on the work of Ford (2006: 81–97) and Bolmsjo et al. (2006: 252–3) let us consider how we can ethically reason to ensure that this restriction of freedom is ethical.

- *Recognize the ethical issue(s)* – Anne is determined to discharge herself but still feels suicidal.
- *Gather the facts and values* – Consider the risks of discharge, look at all the risk factors, considering what is best for Anne (we will explore this in more detail in the next section).
- *Consider the rules* – What do the rules say you should do or not do; look at the relevant professional code, the law and also any relevant policies.
- *Look at any underpinning moral theories* – Relate to the relevant ethical theory, consider the previous section on ethical theory, especially principlism.
- *Consider all options* – It may be that Anne does not want to leave but saying it is a way of communicating her distress, use your therapeutic skills and be person centred.
- *Make a decision and test it* – Confer with your colleagues but also speak to Anne about your decision.
- *Act and reflect on the outcome* – Implement your decision, and then reflect on it in a structured way via the clinical supervision process.

Mental health ethics and values-based practice

A balanced approach to ethical reasoning will work only if the mental health nurse can work with both the facts and the values of a given situation (Ford, 2006; Callaghan, 2009; Fulford, 2009). Thinking ethically within the field of mental health brings its own unique challenges. One such challenge is that conventional approaches to ethics are based on the idea of the rational person in society. However, within the field of mental health the practitioner has to also make sense of the irrational (Fulford et al., 2006). This also brings into play the dimension of power and only within the field of mental health (see Fulford, 2009: 62) 'can a fully conscious adult patient of normal intelligence be treated without consent, not for the protection of others (though this is also possible) but in their own interests'.

That is not to say that because of the presence of irrationality it is not plausible for the mental health nurse to make rational, ethical judgements, it is just that it may be a bit more complex than first thought (Thornton, 2007). As an example, if Anne lacks capacity then using a rational ethical framework such as principlism appears to provide an obvious way forward: protect Anne (principle of beneficence) and therefore act in Anne's best interests (Beauchamp and Childress, 2009; Fulford, 2009). Yet is it really as straightforward as this?

For principlism to work, lacking capacity has to be based on the objective testing of certain cognitive abilities. If all those abilities are not present then a person can be seen to lack capacity and therefore can be seen to not be acting autonomously (Fulford, 2009). Within the field of mental health, judgements regarding capacity tend to be intertwined with diagnostic judgements about the service user's mental disorder. Therefore, for these intertwined judgements to work at a rational and measurable level they need to be based on an objective method of testing, which can lead to complexities (Fulford, 2009). Considering a common mental health symptom such as a delusion, even a standard definition such as one based on the work of Jaspers ([1913] 1997) is subject to different interpretations, to the point that authors such as Oyebode (2008: 122–3) advocate a loose definition that allows an external observer to make a 'situational judgment call'. This means that what were initially perceived as facts, such as mental illness and lack of capacity, are indeed not as objective as first thought and as such are more likely to be value-laden judgements (Roberts, 2004; Cooper, 2009; Fulford, 2009).

Recognizing the value-laden nature of ethical judgements within the field of mental health even when they appear objective allows the mental health nurse the opportunity to consider different viewpoints. As an example, the nurse may consider that protecting Anne (principle of beneficence) is a good thing to do, whereas Anne may see this act as a bad thing because the nurse is controlling and restricting her freedoms (Roberts, 2004; Beauchamp and Childress, 2009; Chodoff, 2009; Fulford, 2009). Principlism does offer a 'reasoned process', however the unique nature of mental health practice means that this reasoned process is not wholly adequate and has its limits, especially when seen from a 'values' perspective (Roberts, 2004; Beauchamp and Childress, 2009; Fulford, 2009).

Woodbridge and Fulford (2004) have developed an approach called value-based practice that assists the mental health nurse to ensure that the ethical reasoning process accounts for the value-laden nature of mental health practice (Cooper, 2009; Fulford, 2009). Values-based practice does not, as a process, focus on 'pre-conceived right outcomes'; instead it focuses on providing a 'good process' for dealing with conflicting values (Fulford, 2009). As an example, Anne's situation viewed through a principlist framework may appear straightforward: protect Anne even if Anne disagrees, especially if Anne lacks capacity. The problem with a straightforward approach is that it is not very person centred, which mental health nurses are required to be (Beauchamp and Childress, 2009; Cooper 2009). However, a values-based approach requires the nurse to work with Anne to understand the presenting values, an understanding which is then used as a starting place to negotiate the way forward (Cooper, 2009).

It is important to note that, for this approach to work, the mental health nurse has to be committed to valuing rights and recovery, collaborative working, and using the best available evidence. For more detail regarding values-based practice see Cooper (2009) and Woodbridge and Fulford (2004). We will now focus on how the skills of values-based practice can assist the mental health nurse during the ethical reasoning process (Ford, 2006; Cooper, 2009; Fulford, 2009). In the previous section on ethical reasoning, step 2 requires the mental health nurses to consider the facts and values. The previous section on ethical theories highlights how they can be used to gather the facts. The following describes how the mental health nurse can also skilfully gather values.

1   Consider Anne's perspective: are Anne's values about the situation being listened to and are they being acted upon?
2   It is important to consider codes of conduct and moral theories, but are these approaches balanced? Have you considered them within the context of Anne's values and narrative?
3   Make sure that Anne's story, while being reframed in the language of science and professionalism, does not lose its person-centred element.
4   Listen to Anne's account of her situation: make sure that this account is fully represented.

Power and abuse

Clearly being ethical is dependent on effective ethical reasoning skills that take into account the value-laden nature of mental health nursing practice, but power is another issue that needs to be taken into account (Roberts, 2004; Chodoff, 2009; Fulford, 2009; Horsfield et al., 2011). The issue of power stems from the use of the mental illness concept: even though the use of this concept is conceptually controversial, it does mean that once an individual is labelled mentally ill the mental health nurse may be sanctioned by society to control that individual (Roberts, 2004; 2005). In part, this approach emanates from the view that an individual who is labelled mentally ill has an increased potential to exhibit diminished judgement and because of this they are then perceived to be potentially more risky or dangerous than the 'average person' in society (Radden, 2002).

The impact of this approach upon mental health nursing practice is that mental health nurses, when therapeutically working with individuals who are labelled as mentally ill, also have to contain and minimize risk (Roberts, 2005; Eales, 2009). In terms of the therapeutic relationship this may mean that an increase in identified risk usually means an increase in the level of control that the mental health nurse exerts over the mental health service user (Roberts, 2005; O'Carroll and Park, 2007). Sometimes this power to control can be explicit, such as the sectioning process, the use of control and restraint, seclusion, locked wards and the covert administration of medicines (Roberts, 2005). However, this power can also be implicit, taking more subtle forms, such as controlling through varying levels of client observations, record keeping, ongoing assessment, planning, implementation and evaluation of 'nursing interventions', individual and group therapy, ongoing risk assessments, regular ward reviews, and so on (Roberts, 2005; Jones and Eales, 2009). The potential downside of the mental health nurse having this power is that even though the therapeutic relationship is intended to be collaborative and person centred the intention in its truest form is dependent on risk, that is the lower the risk the easier it is to not control and therefore be truly collaborative (Roberts, 2005; Perraud et al., 2006).

To ensure that this use of sanctioned power is 'fair and just' the mental health nurse has to practise within a given professional/ethical framework, but as we have seen in the previous section, ethical frameworks do not necessarily take into account the value-laden nature of mental health practice (Roberts, 2005; Thompson et al., 2006; Callaghan, 2009). The concern is that ethical objectivity may be seen as sure defence against abuse in the field of mental health, but if we accept the value-laden nature of the mental health field then abuse can be seen as a real and present danger, and potentially a major ethical issue (Chodoff, 2009; Fulford, 2009).

A further area of concern is that the mental health nurse may be unaware of the implications of using sanctioned power. This lack of awareness may also reflect society's lack of political will to question the power that mental health services hold (Roberts, 2005). The problem with this lack of will is that, as a consequence, 'real ethical issues may be hidden away' (Gomm, 1996).

A starting place for the mental health nurse to address potentially hidden ethical issues when ethically reasoning (see step 2) is to critically reflect on the power relationship they have with a mental health service user. This process of critical reflection is engendered through the use of 'open dialogue' (consider the skills of values-based practice), which focuses on understanding and respecting the service user as a human being rather than as a diagnosis (Roberts, 2005; Ford, 2006; Fulford, 2009). By taking an 'open dialogue' approach the mental health nurse is starting to explore these 'hidden' ethical issues within their practice that they may have been unaware of, such as the coercive impact of psychological interventions (Roberts, 2005; Martinez, 2009). Returning to Anne's case, the use of psychological interventions can be seen to be part of the coercive process which, for Anne, means that her freedoms and choices are restricted by the very treatment she is receiving. Even if choice is available it might have conditions, such as if you comply with treatment (whether you agree with it or not) you are more likely to be discharged (Verkerk et al., 2008).

By engaging Anne in an open dialogue the therapeutic relationship is being given the opportunity to start moving beyond such labels as suicidal and/or severely depressed. It is also moving beyond boxing Anne's experiences into rigid ethical frameworks and is now considering Anne's voice (Roberts, 2005; Anderson and Waters, 2009; Martinez, 2009). The strength of considering Anne's lived experience as part and parcel of the ethical reasoning process is that the mental health nurse can start to use the skills of values-based practice to engender a therapeutic relationship built on true partnership working that is, in turn, potentially less coercive (Borthwick et al., 2001; Roberts, 2005; Ford, 2006; Callaghan, 2009; Cooper, 2009; Fulford, 2009).

Summary of the key points

Mental health nurses have to consider the potential ethical issues that may arise from the use of psychological interventions.

Mental health nurses are professionals who are expected both to know how to act ethically and to do so.

Knowing how to act ethically is based on utilizing the relevant ethical theories, understanding the relevant professional rules, and having the skills to ethically reason.

Mental health nurses, when acting ethically, also have to account for the value-laden nature of mental health care.

Mental health nurses have to consider as an ever-present concern the potential to intentionally or unintentionally abuse their sanctioned powers.

Quick quiz

1 Describe your understanding of the term ethics.
2 Identify the main ethical theories prevalent within the mental health field.
3 Who makes sure mental health nurses are ethical, and how?
4 Which professional rules should mental health nurses follow?
5 Describe, step by step, the ethical reasoning process.
6 What is the difference between a fact and a value?
7 What are the key skills that mental health nurses have to develop in terms of a values-based approach?
8 Identify the two forms of power that exist within mental health nursing care.
9 Define abuse within the field of mental health.
10 Why is looking beyond a diagnostic label so important?

References

Anderson, M. and Waters, K. (2009) Recognition and therapeutic management of self-harm and suicidal behaviour, in P. Callaghan, J. Playle and L. Cooper (eds) *Mental Health Nursing Skills*. Oxford: Oxford University Press.

Barker, P. (2011) Ethics: in search of the good life, in P. Barker (ed.) *Mental Health Ethics: The Human Context*. London: Routledge.

Beauchamp, T.L. and Childress, J.F. (2009) *Principles of Biomedical Ethics*, 6th edn. Oxford: Oxford University Press.

Bloch, S. and Green, S.A. (2009) The scope of psychiatric ethics, in S. Bloch and S.A. Green (eds) *Psychiatric Ethics*, 4th edn. Oxford: Oxford University Press.

Bolmsjo, I.A., Sandman, L. and Andersson, E. (2006) Everyday ethics in the care of elderly people, *Nursing Ethics*, 3(3): 249–63.

Borthwick, A., Holman, C., Kennard, D., McFetridge, M., Messruther, K. and Wilkes, J. (2001) The relevance of moral treatment to contemporary mental health care, in J. Reynolds,

R. Muston, T. Heller, J. Leach, M. McCormick, J. Wallcraft and M. Walsh (eds) *Mental Health Still Matters*. Basingstoke: Palgrave Macmillan.

Callaghan, P. (2009) *Introduction: Mental Nursing Past, Present, and Future,* in P. Callaghan, J. Playle and L. Cooper (eds) *Mental Health Nursing Skills*. Oxford: Oxford University Press.

Chodoff, P. (2009) The abuse of psychiatry, in S. Bloch and S.A. Green (eds) *Psychiatric Ethics,* 4th edn. Oxford: Oxford University Press.

Coady, M. (2009) The nature of professions: implications for psychiatry, in S. Bloch and S.A. Green (eds) *Psychiatric Ethics*, 4th edn. Oxford: Oxford University Press.

Cooper, L. (2009) Values-based mental health nursing practice, in P. Callaghan, J. Playle and L. Cooper (eds) *Mental Health Nursing Skills*. Oxford: Oxford University Press.

Department of Health (DoH) (2006a) *From Values to Action: The Chief Nursing Officer's Review of Mental Health Nursing*. London: Department of Health.

Department of Health (DoH) (2006b) *Best Practice Competencies and Capabilities for Pre-registration Mental Health Nurses in England: The Chief Nursing Officer's Review of Mental Health Nursing*. London: Department of Health.

Eales, S. (2009) Risk assessment and management, in P. Callaghan, J. Playle and L. Cooper (eds) *Mental Health Nursing Skills*. Oxford: Oxford University Press.

Edwards, S.D. (2009) *Nursing Ethics: A Principle-based Approach,* 2nd edn. Basingstoke: Palgrave Macmillan.

Ford, G.G. (2006) *Ethical Reasoning for Mental Health Professionals*. London: Sage Publications.

Fulford, K.W.M. (2009) Values, science and psychiatry, in S. Bloch and S.A. Green (eds) *Psychiatric Ethics,* 4th edn. Oxford: Oxford University Press.

Fulford, K.W.M., Thornton, T. and Graham, G. (2006) *Oxford Textbook of Philosophy and Psychiatry*. Oxford: Oxford University Press.

Gomm, L. (1996) Reversing deviance, in T. Heller, J. Reynolds, R. Gomm, R. Muston and S. Pattison (eds) *Mental Health Matters*. London: Macmillan.

Horsfield, J., Cleary, M., Hunt, G.E. and Walter, G. (2011) Acute care, in P. Barker (ed.) *Mental Health Ethics: The Human Context*. London: Routledge.

Jaspers, K. ([1913] 1997) *General Psychopathology,* trans. J. Hoenig and M.W. Hamilton. Baltimore, MD: Johns Hopkins University Press.

Jones, J. and Eales, S. (2009) Practising safe and effective observation, in P. Callaghan, J. Playle and L. Cooper (eds) *Mental Health Nursing Skills*. Oxford: Oxford University Press.

LaFollette, H. (2000) Introduction, in H. LaFollette (ed.) *The Blackwell Guide to Ethical Theory*. Oxford: Blackwell.

Martinez, R. (2009) Narrative ethics, in S. Bloch and S.A. Green (eds) *Psychiatric Ethics,* 4th edn. Oxford: Oxford University Press.

McKie, A. and Swinton, J. (2000) Community, culture and character: the place of virtues in psychiatric nursing practice, *Journal of Psychiatric and Mental Health Nursing,* 7: 35–42.

Mitchell, V. (2011) Professional relationships, in P. Barker (ed.) *Mental Health Ethics: The Human Context*. London: Routledge.

Nursing and Midwifery Council (NMC) (2008) *The Code: Standards of Conduct, Performance and Ethics for Nurses and Midwives*. London: Nursing and Midwifery Council.

Nursing and Midwifery Council (NMC) (2010) *Standards for Pre-registration Nursing Education*. London: Nursing and Midwifery Council.

O'Carroll, M. and Park, A. (2007) *Essential Mental Health Nursing Skills*. London: Mosby.

Oyebode, F. (2008) *Sims' Symptoms in the Mind: An Introduction to Descriptive Psychopathology*, 4th edn. London: Saunders.

Perraud, S., Delaney, K.R., Carlson-Sabelli, L., Johnson, M.E., Shephard, R. and Paun, O. (2006) Advanced practice psychiatric mental health nursing, finding our core: the therapeutic relationship in 21st century, *Perspectives in Psychiatric Care*, 42(4): 215–26.

Radden, J. (2002) Notes towards a professional ethics for psychiatry, *Australian and New Zealand Journal of Psychiatry*, 36: 52–9.

Roberts, M. (2004) Psychiatric ethics: a critical introduction for mental health nurses, *Journal of Psychiatric and Mental Health Nursing*, 11: 583–8.

Roberts, M. (2005) The production of the psychiatric subject: power, knowledge and Michel Foucault, *Nursing Philosophy*, 6: 33–42.

Scottish Executive (2006) *Rights, Relationships and Recovery: The Report of the National Review of Mental Health Nursing in Scotland*. Edinburgh: Scottish Executive.

Seedhouse, D. (2009) *Ethics: The Heart of Health Care*, 3rd edn. Chichester: John Wiley & Sons.

Smith, K.V. and Godfrey, N.S. (2002) Being a good nurse and doing the right thing: a qualitative study, *Nursing Ethics*, 9(3): 301–12.

Sumner, L.W. (1967) Normative ethics and metaethics, *Ethics*, 77(2): 95–106.

Thompson, I.E., Melia, K.M., Boyd, K.M. and Horsburgh, D. (2006) *Nursing Ethics*, 5th edn. London: Churchill Livingston.

Thornton, T. (2007) *Essential Philosophy of Psychiatry*. Oxford: Oxford University Press.

Verkerk, M., Posltra, L. and de Jonge, M. (2008) Interference in psychiatric care: a sociological and ethical case analysis, in G. Widdershoven, J. MacMillan, J. Hope and L. Van der Scheer (eds) *Empirical Ethics in Psychiatry*. Oxford: Oxford University Press.

Warne, T., McAndrew, S. and Gawthorpe, D. (2011) The mental health nurse, in P. Barker (ed.) *Mental Health Ethics: The Human Context*. London: Routledge.

Woodbridge, K. and Fulford, K.W.M. (2004) *Whose Values? A Workbook for Values-based Practice in Mental Health Care*. London: Sainsbury Centre for Mental Health.

Conclusion: psychological interventions and the mental health nurse's future development

Grahame Smith

Chapter aim and objectives

Aim

*   To explore the key themes articulated in the book while considering how these themes impact upon the mental health nurse's future development.

Objectives

*   To summarize the journey so far and to provide a chapter-by-chapter overview.
*   To identify how the newly qualified nurse can continue to develop their practice.
*   To analyse the notions of lifelong learning, expert practice and critical reflection.

A summary of the book

The intention of this concluding chapter is, first, to summarize the learning journey so far, and then to look at how the newly qualified mental health nurse can continue to develop skilfully in their future use of psychological interventions.

The introductory chapter highlights the importance of collaboration, the impact of risk and the need to make sense of the underpinning evidence; these themes also run throughout the book. This chapter captures the importance of listening and responding to the service user in a way that moves beyond professional assumptions: 'It should be the primary function of the mental health nurse to develop the capacity for listening and responding to the patient and their own interpretations of their internal and external worlds, rather than providing them with a professionally orientated "map of reality"' (Warne and McAndrew, 2007: 227).

Chapter 2 explores the use of these communication skills in more depth, but it has to be acknowledged that sometimes it feels difficult to use these skills effectively within the field of mental health when managing risk. To help, Chapter 1 provides a useful insight into the management of risk; this chapter links to Chapter 11 which looks at risk and also power in terms of how they can be framed within a 'good process'. The intention of these chapters is to assist the mental health student nurse:

> To practice in a manner that seeks to promote understanding through 'reciprocal elucidation' therefore is to engage in an ongoing and open-ended process. It is to understand that psychiatric discourses, categorizations and presuppositions are historically and politically constituted, and it is to be willing to subject them to critical reflection and questioning, while also allowing clients to be legitimate participants in that dialogue.
>
> (Roberts, 2005: 40)

Chapters 3 to 10 build on this intention but they also provide a good grounding in the use of psychological interventions (Department of Health, 2006b; Callaghan, 2009; Nursing and Midwifery Council, 2010). Of course, these chapters do not deal with every situation a student mental health nurse may face during their pre-registration training; rather, they aim to complement your training experiences by giving practical examples of how psychological interventions can be used in a variety of settings and contexts. On this basis this chapter will explore how the knowledge and skills accrued both from your training and from this book can then be further developed as you make the transition from student nurse to qualified practitioner. This transition can be a difficult time: 'It has been widely recognised that newly qualified nurses in the UK experience a period of transition and change from being a student to working as a staff nurse. This transition period has been identified as a stressful experience' (Higgins et al., 2010: 508). But there is light at the end of the tunnel and certainly preceptorship programmes can be both useful and helpful:

> As I took up my first nursing post I had the same anxieties that I experienced as a student – my flatmate's sleeping pattern suffered in the first week as I was so nervous that I could not sleep. How will other staff and patients see me? Am I expected to know every thing? What if I make a mistake? Will I be liked? Can I do justice to the profession? Newly qualified staff need to feel they can voice these kinds of concerns and communicate their anxieties with members of the team, and without feeling they are incompetent or are expected lo know everything. Becoming part of a team and settling in takes time and working shifts means that it takes a while to meet everyone. The trust where I took my first job operated a preceptorship policy so that I was supernumerary for a period of time with a mentor assigned to work with me. Preceptorship normally lasts around six months and incorporates development and support for the newly qualified nurse.
>
> (Pearson, 2009: 32)

While acknowledging the potential anxieties of the newly qualified nurse this chapter will now focus on exploring in more depth the need for the qualified mental health nurse to actively engage in continuously developing their practice, which includes the delivery of psychological interventions (Department of Health, 2006a; Nursing and Midwifery Council, 2008b).

Looking to the future

Psychological interventions are a key component in the process of assisting a service user towards recovery but using psychological interventions effectively in practice is not always easy for the newly qualified mental health nurse, especially when there are other clinical factors present which the mental health nurse may not have direct control over, such as good housing and employment (Brimblecombe et al., 2007; Finfgeld-Connett, 2008; Callaghan, 2009; Norman and Ryrie, 2009). On this basis the newly qualified mental health nurse has to quickly recognize that psychological interventions are situated in a holistic and complex clinical picture where the mental health nurse not only has to be appropriately skilled in the use of psychological interventions, but also on behalf of the service user they have to be able to effectively influence external agencies and the wider community (Brimblecombe et al., 2007; Finfgeld-Connett, 2008; Callaghan, 2009). Additionally, the field of mental health nursing is constantly changing, challenging the mental health nurse to deal with constant change while needing to deliver high-quality care to service users who have complex needs (Crowe and O'Malley, 2006; Norman and Ryrie, 2009).

To ensure that the mental health nurse is adaptive to change and can also deliver high-quality care, the mental health nurse needs not only to have a full set of baseline skills but also continue to develop and enhance their skills as part of a 'lifelong learning journey' (Paley and Shapiro, 2001; Fox, 2009). As mentioned in the introductory chapter a mental health nurse's knowledge is accrued through their pre-qualifying training; this knowledge is then developed into 'ways of knowing' which the qualified mental health nurse then further develops through their own practice experiences (Carper, 1978; Welsh and Lyons, 2001; Hardy et al., 2002; Department of Health, 2006a; 2006b). Practice-orientated knowledge (expert practice) is underpinned by scientific evidence and uses evidence situated within the mental health nurse–service user relationship, which should sensitively reflect the specific needs of the mental health service user (Benner and Tanner, 1987; Welsh and Lyons, 2001; Franks, 2004; Finfgeld-Connett, 2008; Callaghan and Crawford, 2009).

Developing expert practice is part and parcel of the mental health nurse's lifelong learning journey where expert mental health nurses not only have expert practice skills, but are also able to deal with ambiguous and complex clinical situations where the outcome is not always certain (Finfgeld-Connett, 2008). Key to being an expert mental health nurse is the need for the nurse to be self-aware at a level at which they are able to understand their own strengths and areas for further development, in other words they have to be skilled in critical reflection (Crowe and O'Malley, 2006; Finfgeld-Connett, 2008).

Being skilled in critical reflection, is, in part, about being able to think critically while also creating the opportunity to reflect on everyday work situations in a structured way (Gould and Masters, 2004; Fox, 2009). Reflective practice requires the mental health nurse to be a rational and logical thinker but they must also be able to work with any underlying beliefs, values and assumptions (Crowe and O'Malley, 2006; O'Carroll and Park, 2007).

To summarize, the onus on the newly qualified mental health nurse is to continue to develop the quality and effectiveness of the psychological interventions they deliver by engaging in a lifelong learning journey. On this basis the following sections will explore the journey in more depth by specifically exploring the notions of lifelong learning, expert practice and critical reflection.

Lifelong learning

Lifelong learning is a concept that is used often but there is generally not an accepted definition, on this basis this section takes a broad view of lifelong learning which is seen as a holistic process of developing skills and understanding (Sharples, 2000; Tuijnman and Bostrom, 2002; Nursing and Midwifery Council, 2008a; Fox, 2009; Kedge and Appleby, 2009). The process is also viewed as learning across the lifespan of an individual and it includes learning outside such formal settings as educational institutions and programmes (Tuijnman and Bostrom, 2002). The impact for post-qualified mental health nurses is that there is an expectation, led by employers and the professional body, that the mental health nurse will keep their skills and knowledge up to date throughout their working life (Nursing and Midwifery Council, 2008a; Fox, 2009; Kedge and Appleby, 2009).

In this context lifelong learning becomes entwined with the need for the nurse to engage in a process of 'continuous professional development' on which basis the Nursing and Midwifery Council (NMC) provides a set of standards for post-registration education and practice (PREP) (Nursing and Midwifery Council, 2008b; Kedge and Appleby, 2009). PREP assists the mental health nurse to keep up to date with new developments in practice, to continue to develop their practice and it also aims to 'encourage the nurse to think and reflect' (Nursing and Midwifery Council, 2008b: 3).

To have value within a work context, lifelong learning needs to link to a reflective process where the nurse can explore, appreciate and develop their life's experiences (Eason, 2010). According to Welsh and Lyons (2001: 299) mental health nurses occupy a unique position within mental health practice in that it is the mental health nurse who 'usually has the greatest amount of direct mental health service user contact'. It is this unique position that shapes the knowledge the mental health nurse needs, which is usually further developed by a process of reflecting and acting upon those reflections (Welsh and Lyons, 2001; Finfgeld-Connett, 2008).

Reflection and understanding their practice is an important part of the nurse's journey towards being an expert (Finfgeld-Connett, 2008). As this journey is unique to each nurse, and as each nurse's experiences are unique and dynamic, the learning process needs to take this into account (Finfgeld-Connett, 2008). This does not mean that more generalized learning such as formal education has no part to play, but as there is a focus on the mental health nurse using their unique practice experiences to improve the care they subsequently deliver, then more informal methods of learning need also to be utilized (Benner, 1982; Kuiper and Pesut, 2004; Eason, 2010). Benner makes the following point about expertise and experience, which will be explored further in the next section.

> At the expert level, the performer no longer relies on an analytical principle (rule, guideline, maxim) to connect her/his understanding of the situation to an appropriate action. The expert nurse, with her/his enormous back-ground of experience, has an intuitive grasp of the situation and zeros in on the accurate region of the problem without wasteful consideration of a large range of unfruitful possible problem situations.
>
> (Benner, 1982: 405)

Expert practice

A paper by Jasper makes the point that;

> Although the term 'expert' is used commonly in nursing practice and the nursing literature, it is apparent from this analysis and subsequent discussion that the term is ambiguous and difficult to clarify. The attribution of expertise remains linked to subjective criteria and reputation, with all of the defining attributes (knowledge, experience, pattern recognition and recognition by others) having loosely defined parameters.
>
> (Jasper, 1994: 775)

Taking on board Jasper's position, this section will not aim to define the notion of the expert nurse; rather it will explore how expertise fits within the mental health nurse's lifelong learning journey. According to Finfgeld-Connett (2008) expert nurses are 'sculptured' by formal education, but time and experience are needed to apply the finishing touches. The process of being sculptured starts with the foundation knowledge that the mental health nurse accrues from their pre-registration training experiences (Welsh and Lyons, 2001). On qualifying, the mental health nurse will possess knowledge from the human and physical sciences combined with a wide range of interpersonal skills (Welsh and Lyons, 2001; Department of Health, 2006b; Norman and Ryrie, 2009). This knowledge and wide range of skills are then further developed by the nurse's own experience of being a practitioner (Welsh and Lyons, 2001; Hardy et al., 2002). Benner (1982), based on the then unpublished work of Dreyfus and Dreyfus, proposed what is now a seminal description of the expert nurse's learning journey;

1. Novice – learning to be a nurse
2. Advanced Beginner – starting to contextualise theories via practical experience
3. Competent – can manage most standard clinical situations but lacks speed and flexibility

4   Proficient – Looks at situations holistically, can recognise non-standard situations

5   Expert – not just reliant on rules to manage situations, can also use tacit knowledge

(Benner, 1982: 403–6)

Both expert and newly qualified mental health nurses will be able to cope with a range of situations, but where the newly qualified nurse will lack some 'speed and flexibility' the expert nurse is not only more 'analytical and fluid' but they can also recognize and skilfully deal with an unexpected clinical situation (Finfgeld-Connett, 2008; Lyneham et al., 2008). This ability to effectively handle uncertain, and also complex, clinical situations is based on the expert nurse not using just scientific knowledge, but also being able to use tacit knowledge (see the introductory chapter) (Finfgeld-Connett, 2008). Key to using different forms of knowing is the ability to be self-aware whilst also being committed to engage in the process of reflecting on practice (Welsh and Lyons, 2001; Hardy et al., 2002; Finfgeld-Connett, 2008; Lyneham et al., 2008).

Critical reflection

Being able to engage in reflection or reflecting on action, is both a professional requirement and a supportive component of making effective clinical decisions and judgements (Schon, 1983; Welsh and Lyons, 2001; Kuiper and Pesut, 2004; Moloney and Hahessy, 2006). On this basis, reflection (see also Chapter 2) is a process which requires the mental health nurse to not only re-examine their practice experiences, but also to focus on changing their practice for the better, meaning that they need to action plan and then act upon this plan (Smith and Johnston, 2002; Gould and Masters, 2004). To be an effective thinking process, reflection needs to be both structured and critical (Smith and Johnston, 2002; Gould and Masters, 2004; Kedge and Appleby, 2009).

Rather than focus on a model of structured reflection (there are a number of good texts dedicated to this subject), this section will concentrate on how to think critically during the process of reflection. Reflective skills are taught in undergraduate pre-registration mental health nursing programmes, first at a descriptive level and, then, as the student moves through their programme of study they are increasingly encouraged to be more critically reflective (Crowe and O'Malley, 2006; Department of Health, 2006b). A key part of being critically reflective is to be able to identify critical incidents that arise from your practice experience. You then need to engage in a process of questioning and re-questioning your actions. Any assumptions need to be challenged (Gould and Masters, 2004; Crowe and O'Malley, 2006). Based on a paper by Crowe and O'Malley (2006) the following list provides a few examples of the types of question you might ask:

- What is happening currently and what is problematic about it?
- What rationales are provided for the current practice/situation?
- What are the social, cultural, political and historical factors that underpin the development and maintenance of this practice?

- How does the practice/situation impact on the consumer?
- What are the options for potential alternative actions?
- What are the rationales that support alternative options? What might you further need to know? What does the research, literature and other resources say about the issues/options?

(Crowe and O'Malley, 2006: 85)

Once qualified, the mental health nurse, who will be a practitioner in their own right, will be expected to continue to engage in this thorough and systematic examination of their practice. The most common method will be through the process of clinical supervision (Crowe and O'Malley, 2006; Department of Health, 2006a; Moloney and Hahessy, 2006; Brimblecombe et al., 2007; Freshwater, 2011). It is also important to recognize that critical reflection is a skill and it takes time to develop, especially where the skill is used by the nurse to both learn from practice and also to improve the quality of care the nurse delivers (Crowe and O'Malley, 2006; Moloney and Hahessy, 2006; Jasper and Rolfe, 2011).

A final point

While it is professionally important for the mental health nurse to engage in a life-long learning journey that is explicitly linked with the notion of being an expert, this needs to be tempered with the following words of caution: 'For some nurses their perceived level of expertise, the theoretical knowledge and personal knowing, will lead to a heightened sense of power and of being in control, which in turn promotes self-confidence, albeit a somewhat false confidence' (Warne and McAndrew, 2007: 227). To avoid this happening the mental health nurse needs to remember the point articulated in the introductory chapter of how important it is to ground the use of psychological interventions in a way that is collaborative and person-centred (Bracken and Thomas, 2005; Hamilton and Roper, 2006; Department of Health, 2006a; Simpson 2009).

Summary of the key points

Mental health nurses, when delivering psychological interventions, should also consider such issues as the importance of collaboration, the impact of risk and the need to make sense of the underpinning evidence.
Mental health nurses are required to professionally engage with lifelong learning through the process of PREP.
A key tenet of expert mental health nursing practice is the need to learn from practice through the process of reflection.
Being critically reflective is a skill that the mental health nurse is required to develop while acknowledging that it takes practice and time.

Quick quiz

1   What was your most useful chapter(s)?
2   Define lifelong learning.
3   What is PREP?
4   Describe the stages of the expert nurse.
5   What differentiates an expert nurse from a competent nurse?
6   To be effective what does reflection need to be?
7   What role does 'questioning' play in the reflective process?
8   Describe a common form of reflection.

References

Benner, P. (1982) From novice to expert, *American Journal of Nursing*, 82(3): 402–7.

Benner, P. and Tanner, C. (1987) Clinical judgment: how expert nurses use intuition, *American Journal of Nursing*, 87(1): 23–31.

Bracken, P. and Thomas, P. (2005) *Postpsychiatry: Mental Health in a Postmodern World.* Oxford: Oxford University Press.

Brimblecombe, N., Tingle, A., Tunmore, R. and Murrell, T. (2007) Implementing holistic practices in mental health nursing: a national consultation, *International Journal of Nursing Studies*, 44: 339–48.

Callaghan, P. (2009) Introduction: mental nursing past, present, and future, in P. Callaghan, J. Playle and L. Cooper (eds) *Mental Health Nursing Skills*. Oxford: Oxford University Press.

Callaghan, P. and Crawford, P. (2009) Evidence-based mental health nursing practice, in P. Callaghan, J. Playle and L. Cooper (eds) (2009) *Mental Health Nursing Skills*. Oxford: Oxford University Press.

Carper, B.A. (1978) Fundamental patterns of knowing in nursing, *Advances in Nursing Science*, 1(1): 13–23.

Crowe, M.T. and O'Malley, J. (2006) Teaching critical reflection skills for advanced mental health nursing practice: a deconstructive–reconstructive approach, *Journal of Advanced Nursing*, 56(1): 79–87.

Department of Health (2006a) *From Values to Action: The Chief Nursing Officer's Review of Mental Health Nursing.* London: Department of Health.

Department of Health (2006b) *Best Practice Competencies and Capabilities for Pre-registration Mental Health Nurses in England: The Chief Nursing Officer's Review of Mental Health Nursing.* London: Department of Health.

Eason, T. (2010) Lifelong learning: fostering a culture of curiosity, *Creative Nursing*, 16(4): 155–9.

Finfgeld-Connett, D. (2008) Concept synthesis of the art of nursing, *Journal of Advanced Nursing*, 62(3): 381–8.

Fox, C. (2009) Personal and professional development, in P. Callaghan, J. Playle and L. Cooper (eds) *Mental Health Nursing Skills*. Oxford: Oxford University Press.

Franks, V. (2004) Evidence-based uncertainty in mental health nursing, *Journal of Psychiatric and Mental Health Nursing*, 11: 99–105.

Freshwater, M. (2011) Clinical supervision and reflective practice, in G. Rolfe, M. Jasper and D. Freshwater (eds) *Critical Reflection in Practice: Generating Knowledge for Care*, 2nd edn. Basingstoke: Palgrave Macmillan.

Gould, B. and Masters, H. (2004) Learning to make sense: the use of critical incident analysis in facilitated reflective groups of mental health student nurses, *Learning in Health and Social Care*, 3(2): 53–63.

Hamilton, B. and Roper, C. (2006) Troubling 'insight': power and possibilities in mental health care, *Journal of Psychiatric and Mental Health Nursing*, 13: 416–22.

Hardy, S., Garbett, R., Titchen, A. and Manley, K. (2002) Exploring nursing expertise: nurses talk nursing, *Nursing Inquiry*, 9: 196–202.

Higgins, G., Spencer, R.L. and Kane, R. (2010) A systematic review of the experiences and perceptions of the newly qualified nurse in the United Kingdom, *Nurse Education Today*, 30: 499–508.

Jasper, M. (1994) Expert: a discussion of the implications of the concept as used in nursing, *Journal of Advanced Nursing*, 20: 769–76.

Jasper, M. and Rolfe, G. (2011) Critical reflection and the emergence of professional knowledge, in G. Rolfe, M. Jasper and D. Freshwater (2011) *Critical Reflection in Practice: Generating Knowledge for Care*, 2nd edn. Basingstoke: Palgrave Macmillan.

Kedge, S. and Appleby, B. (2009) Promoting a culture of curiosity within nursing practice, *British Journal of Nursing*, 18(10): 635–7.

Kuiper, R.A. and Pesut, D.J. (2004) Promoting cognitive and metacognitive reflective reasoning skills in nursing practice: self-regulated learning theory, *Journal of Advanced Nursing*, 45(4): 381–91.

Lyneham, J., Parkinson, C. and Denholm, C. (2008) Explicating Benner's concept of expert practice: intuition in emergency nursing, *Journal of Advanced Nursing*, 64(4): 380–7.

Moloney, J. and Hahessy, S. (2006) Using reflection in everyday orthopaedic nursing practice, *Journal of Orthopaedic Nursing*, 10: 49–55.

Norman, I. and Ryrie, I. (2009) Future directions: taking recovery into society, in I. Norman and I. Ryrie (eds) *The Art and Science of Mental Health Nursing: A Textbook of Principles and Practice*, 2nd edn. Maidenhead: McGraw-Hill.

Nursing and Midwifery Council (2008a) *The Code: Standards of Conduct, Performance and Ethics for Nurses and Midwives*. London: Nursing and Midwifery Council.

Nursing and Midwifery Council (2008b) *The Prep Handbook*. London: Nursing and Midwifery Council.

Nursing and Midwifery Council (2010) *Standards for Pre-registration Nursing Education*. London: Nursing and Midwifery Council.

O'Carroll, M. and Park, A. (2007) *Essential Mental Health Nursing Skills*. London: Mosby.

Paley, G. and Shapiro, D. (2001) Evidence-based psychological interventions in mental health nursing, *Nursing Times*, 97(3): 34.

Pearson, H. (2009) Transition from nursing student to staff nurse: a personal reflection, *Paediatric Nursing*, 21(3): 30–2.

Roberts, M. (2005) The production of the psychiatric subject: power, knowledge and Michel Foucault, *Nursing Philosophy*, 6: 33–42.

Schon, D. (1983) From technical rationality to reflection-in-action, in R. Harrison, F. Reeve, A. Hanson and J. Clarke (eds) *Supporting Lifelong Learning: Perspectives on Learning*. London: RoutledgeFalmer.

Sharples, M. (2000) The design of personal mobile technologies for lifelong learning, *Computers and Education*, 34: 177–93.

Simpson, A. (2009) Working in partnership, in P. Callaghan, J. Playle and L. Cooper (eds) *Mental Health Nursing Skills*. Oxford: Oxford University Press.

Smith, B. and Johnston, Y. (2002) Using structured clinical preparation to stimulate reflection and foster critical thinking, *Journal of Nursing Education*, 41(4): 182–5.

Tuijnman, A. and Bostrom, A. (2002) Changing notions of lifelong education and lifelong learning, *International Review of Education*, 48(1/2): 93–110.

Warne, T. and McAndrew, S. (2007) Passive patient or engaged expert? Using a Ptolemaic approach to enhance mental health nurse education and practice, *International Journal of Mental Health Nursing*, 16: 224–9.

Welsh, I. and Lyons, C.M. (2001) Evidence-based care and the case for intuition and tacit knowledge in clinical assessment and decision making in mental health nursing practice: an empirical contribution to the debate, *Journal of Psychiatric and Mental Health Nursing*, 8: 299–305.

Index

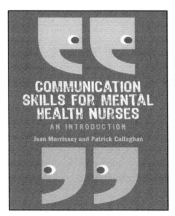

COMMUNICATION SKILLS FOR MENTAL HEALTH NURSES

Jean Morrissey and Patrick Callaghan

9780335238705 (Paperback)
2011

eBook also available

This new mental health nursing text is a practical guide to the core communication skills and interventions used in mental health. Designed as an introduction, the book examines key elements of the therapeutic relationship, covering different core aspects of practice including solution focused interventions and motivational interviewing in mental health practice.

Key features:

- Packed full of clinical case studies, activities, examples and points for reflection
- Covers core areas of the therapeutic relationship including: reflecting on self, the value of small talk, being supportive, asking questions, giving information, building confidence and resolving conflict
- Enables readers to try out techniques and hone their communication skills in practice

www.openup.co.uk

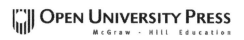

OPEN UNIVERSITY PRESS
McGraw - Hill Education

MENTAL HEALTH NURSING CASE BOOK

Nick Wrycraft

9780335242955 (Paperback)
September 2012

eBook also available

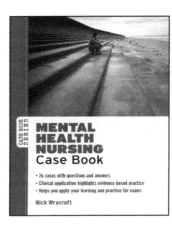

This case book is aimed at mental health nursing students and those going into mental health settings, such as social workers. The cases include a wide range of mental health diagnoses from common problems such as anxiety or depression through to severe and enduring conditions such as schizophrenia. The cases will be organised into sections by life stage from childhood through to old age.

Key features:

- Uses a case study approach which provides a realistic context that students will find familiar
- Each case study will commence with a practice focused scenario
- Provides a commentary offering insights, perspectives and references to theories, research and further explanations and discussion

www.openup.co.uk

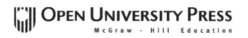
OPEN UNIVERSITY PRESS
McGraw · Hill Education

14716536R00107

Printed in Great Britain
by Amazon.co.uk, Ltd.,
Marston Gate.